Clinical Cases in Fluid and Electrolyte Balance

An Acute Care Approach

Dr Geoffrey Couser dedicates this work with love to his children, Thomas and Grace, who every day teach him what education is really all about.

Clinical Cases in Fluid and Electrolyte Balance

An Acute Care Approach

DR GEOFFREY A COUSER
ASSOCIATE PROFESSOR JUSTIN T WALLS

The *McGraw·Hill* Companies

Sydney New York San Francisco Auckland
Bangkok Bogotá Caracas Hong Kong
Kuala Lumpur Lisbon London Madrid
Mexico City Milan New Delhi San Juan
Seoul Singapore Taipei Toronto

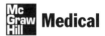 **Medical**

First published 2009

Text, illustrations and design © 2009 McGraw-Hill Australia Pty Ltd

National Library of Australia Cataloguing-in-Publication Data
Author: Couser, Geoffrey A.
Title: Clinical cases in fluid and electrolyte balance: an acute care approach / Geoffrey A Couser, Justin T. Walls.
ISBN: 9780070165625 (pbk.)
Series: Clinical cases.
Notes: Includes index, Bibliography.
Subjects: Emergency medicine, Water-electrolyte balance (Physiology), Water-electrolyte imbalances, Body fluid disorders, Medical technology.
Other Authors/Contributors: Walls, Justin T., 1967-
Dewey Number: 616.39

Published in Australia by
McGraw-Hill Australia Pty Ltd
Level 2, 82 Waterloo Road, North Ryde NSW 2113

1006088780

Publisher: Elizabeth Walton
Managing Editor: Kathryn Fairfax
Editor: Elaine Cochrane
Editorial Co-ordinator: Fiona Richardson
Art Director: Astred Hicks
Design: Jan Schmoeger, Designpoint
Proofreader: Kim Ross
Indexer: Glenda Brown
Typeset in India by codeMantra
Printed in China on 80 gsm woodfree by 1010 Printing International Ltd

The McGraw·Hill Companies

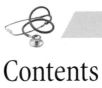

Contents

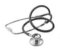

About the authors

Dr Geoffrey A Couser MBBS FACEM GradCert ULT

Department of Emergency Medicine, Royal Hobart Hospital
Liverpool Street, Hobart, Tasmania 7000
geoffrey.couser@dhhs.tas.gov.au

Geoff is a consultant emergency physician at the Royal Hobart Hospital, and a clinical senior lecturer at the University of Tasmania. He has designed and implemented workplace-based programs for both undergraduates and postgraduates. He is the section editor for education and training for the journal *Emergency Medicine Australasia*. Together with Associate Professor Justin Walls, he is a director of Biomedical Education Australia, an integrated clinical education and health science consultancy that provides educational services to educational institutions and workplaces.

Associate Professor Justin T Walls PhD DipMedEd

Faculty of Health Science
University of Tasmania
Private Bag 24
Hobart, Tasmania 7001
j.walls@utas.edu.au

Justin is currently the Associate Dean Teaching and Learning in the Faculty of Health Science at the University of Tasmania and has an extensive research and teaching background in systems physiology. He has gained postgraduate qualifications in medical education at the University of Dundee. He is responsible for the organisation and delivery of key medical and health science units and is playing a key role in the design and implementation of a new five-year undergraduate medical curriculum at the University of Tasmania.

Acknowledgments

All clinical photographs, X-rays and electrocardiograms were provided by Dr Geoffrey Couser. Consent has been obtained from patients for use where identifying features are included.

The authors would like to thank Associate Professor David Johns for his advice and guidance in relation to the respiratory physiology and specifically his input to the spirometry testing material in the text.

Dr Geoffrey Couser's work was partly supported by an educational grant from the Royal Hobart Hospital Education and Training Committee.

Introduction

Hospital staff frequently prescribe intravenous fluid therapy and order pathology tests, and most patients admitted to hospital receive intravenous therapy or have some pathological investigation performed. Although intravenous fluid therapy is not without its complications, its prescription is usually left to the most junior of staff. Pathology testing accounts for a significant and growing proportion of the annual health budget; so it is essential that practitioners understand how to use and interpret the most basic tests appropriately.

This book aims to present common clinical cases that combine the practice of emergency medicine with the fundamental biomedical science behind fluid, electrolyte and acid–base balance, thereby enabling the reader to obtain a deeper understanding of their role and to appreciate the importance of the biomedical science to everyday practice. Health science students will see the science in action and how the often esoteric topics of fluid and electrolyte balance have a practical application. More advanced students and practitioners can review the cases and revise the biomedical science topics in the context of their own clinical experience. Combining the biomedical science with clinical practice can lead to a deeper learning experience in both spheres for learners at all levels.

This is not a comprehensive text on the clinical conditions discussed or the basic science behind them—readers may wish to refer to definitive texts in emergency medicine or physiology to obtain a more in-depth coverage of the topics—but this book provides a vital link between the clinical and the biomedical science. Each informs the other.

Intravenous fluids

Intravenous fluids are commonly prescribed in emergency departments, and it is essential for staff to understand indications for their use.

Fluids are commonly prescribed for volume replacement, rehydration and resuscitation, and for the administration of antibiotics and other medication. They are invariably used in the pre-operative and post-operative period (when significant disorders can arise), and are often prescribed on an empirical basis; that is, a fixed volume is prescribed over a fixed time without any ongoing assessment of whether it is too little or too much for the individual patient.

A number of complications can arise from either too much or too little fluid replacement, with hyponatraemia being a common complication in hospitals. In general, it is best to avoid administering intravenous fluid if there is a more suitable alternative, such as if the patient can rehydrate by the oral or nasogastric route, or can take medications orally.

There are a number of fluids available for use; these are detailed in Table I.1 overleaf. All have their indications and complications, and clinicians need to be aware of these before prescribing their use. The use of a number of these fluids will be presented in the cases that follow, and the different indications and contraindications for each will be considered.

Significantly, each hospital has its own protocols and policies concerning intravenous fluids and the management of different conditions. This book is not meant to be a definitive resource—users must refer to local staff and the guidelines of the hospital concerned.

Osmolarity, osmolality and equivalents

These terms are frequently used when referring to commonly used intravenous fluids, but are often poorly understood or used incorrectly. The osmolarity of a solution is simply a count of the number of dissolved particles and is a measure of the effective gradient for water movement assuming that all the solute is completely impermeant. The plasma osmolarity of a solution is less than osmolality, because the total plasma weight (used to calculate osmolality) excludes the weight of any solutes, while the total plasma volume (used to calculate osmolarity) includes solute content. Both terms are often used interchangeably as there is little difference between the absolute values. The equivalent (Eq or eq) is a common measurement unit used when discussing body fluid balance. An equivalent of an electrolyte is the amount that produces 1 mole of positive or negative charges when it dissolves. Equivalents therefore provide a means of quantifying the number of available charges in a solution rather than the number of dissolved particles that molarity refers to.

Electrolytes

Electrolyte disorders are both a common cause and a common effect of hospital admission, yet medical and nursing staff continue to have difficulty

Table I.1 Comparison of commonly used intravenous fluids

Solution	Common name	Osmolality (mOsmol/L)	Sodium equivalent (mequiv/L)	Osmolality (compared to plasma)	Tonicity (with reference to cell membrane)
Sodium chloride 0.9%	Normal saline	308	154	Isosmolar	Isotonic
Sodium chloride 0.45%	Half normal saline	154	77	Hyposmolar	Hypotonic
Sodium chloride 0.45% and glucose 5%	Five and a half	432	75	Hyperosmolar	Hypotonic
Glucose 5%		278	–	Isosmolar	Hypotonic
Glucose 10%		555	–	Hyperosmolar	Hypotonic
Sodium chloride 0.18% and glucose 4%	Four and a fifth	284	31	Isosmolar	Hypotonic
Hartmann's solution	Hartmann's/ lactated Ringer's	278	131	Isosmolar	Isotonic
Human albumin solution 4.5%		275	100–160	Isosmolar	Isotonic

understanding them. A proper understanding of the significance of disorders of sodium and potassium in a clinical environment requires a working knowledge of the different fluid compartments in the body and how they interact. This means that a review of the biomedical science is essential, and readers are referred to further reading resources at the end of each chapter.

Acid–base balance

Acid–base disorders are found in many patients who present to emergency departments, and venous blood samples are frequently used in departmental blood gas machines to obtain an immediate electrolyte and haemoglobin result. Venous blood results have been shown to provide information as accurate as arterial blood. Understanding and interpretation of acid–base results can guide therapy and provide a rapid assessment of the severity of illness. Blood gases are used frequently in the cases that follow, and understanding the biomedical science behind them can greatly assist diagnosis and management.

How to use the cases

Readers are encouraged to put themselves into the role of a junior doctor in the emergency department of a public hospital. It's busy, but there's always an emergency physician nearby to whom you can present your patients. The cases are presented in an undifferentiated and problem-focused format, just as 'real' patients are when they present to a hospital.

Each case begins with a list of clinical and physiology learning objectives detailing what students can be expected to know by the end of the chapter. It may be best, however, to refer to the objectives after reading the case, as a number of clues are unavoidably contained within them, thus spoiling one of the advantages of learning by using undifferentiated conditions. The story unfolds around a timeline, with information being presented as it would be in 'real time'. Clinical questions are inserted at appropriate times to encourage

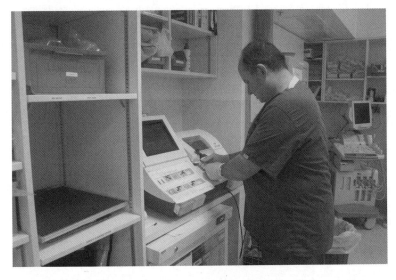

Dr Geoff Couser using the blood gas machine at the Royal Hobart Hospital

the reader to make decisions and to consider the next appropriate course of action. The answers are provided, but you should not read them until after you have considered the answer yourself. Pathology and radiological results are presented to be interpreted, with reference ranges as per the *Royal College of Pathologists Australia Manual*; these have been adjusted for age and gender. Each case has an epilogue and a summary of useful tips.

Even though each case stands alone and can be read individually, it is important to recognise that the underlying concepts are built upon sequentially throughout the book. Readers will find it valuable to review cases in chronological order, as the progressive presentation of concepts will aid understanding.

Each case has a series of self-assessment questions designed to suit differing levels of knowledge. Each case is referenced with landmark papers that provide more in-depth coverage of the relevant topic. Finally, the appendix consists of a curriculum map of the cases where the key clinical and science topics are listed and can be easily identified as a reference.

References and further reading

1   Grocott, M.P.W., Mythen, M.G. & Gan, T.J. Perioperative fluid management and clinical outcomes in adults. *Anesth Analg* 2005; 100: 1093–1106.

2   Hilton, A.K., Pellegrino, V.A. & Scheinkestel, C.D. Avoiding common problems associated with intravenous fluid therapy. *MJA* 2008; 189: 509–513.

3   Lin, M., Liu, S.J. & Lim, I.T. Disorders of water imbalance. *Emerg Med Clin N Am* 2005; 23: 749–770.

4   Middleton, P., Kelly, A.M., Brown, J., & Robertson, M. Agreement between arterial and central venous values for pH, bicarbonate, base excess, and lactate. *Emerg Med J* Aug 2006; 23 (8): 622–624.

5   Molyneux, E.M. & Maitland, K. Intravenous fluids—getting the balance right. *N Engl J Med* 2005; 353 (9): 941–944.

6   The Royal College of Pathologists of Australasia, *Royal College of Pathologists Australia RCPA Manual*, 4th edn, RCPA, Surry Hills, 2004.

7   Shafiee, M.A.S., Bohn, D., Hoorn, E.J. & Halperin, M.L. How to select optimal maintenance intravenous fluid therapy. *Q J Med* 2003; 96: 601–610.

Case 1
Julia was feeling woozy …

A teenage girl presents to the emergency department feeling faint. Your assessment and management of this common problem must identify any serious underlying pathology, if present, and begin appropriate management.

Clinical learning objectives

- Understand what is meant by the term 'syncope'.
- Describe the issues to consider when assessing a patient presenting with syncope.
- Know how to utilise bedside, laboratory and radiological investigations correctly when you are assessing a patient presenting with syncope or 'pre-syncope'.
- Be able to use established clinical pathways to differentiate between benign and potentially dangerous causes of syncope.

Physiology learning objectives

- Describe how posture can influence blood pressure in the hypovolaemic patient.
- Outline the interrelationships between total body water, intracellular fluid and extracellular fluid.
- Describe what is meant by the terms dehydration and hypovolaemia.
- Describe the role of the kidney in maintaining body fluid and electrolyte homeostasis.
- Understand the importance of assessing hydration state before reviewing electrolyte values.
- Define what is meant by diuresis and discuss the mechanism by which thiazide diuretic use may lead to increased water, Na, Cl and K loss from the body.

Timeline

09:53	Julia presents to emergency department, triaged category 4.
10:32	Collapses in waiting room, brought into an emergency department cubicle and the nursing assessment begins.
10:40	Vital signs recorded, 12-lead ECG completed, intern commences assessment.
12:30	Blood results available.
12:45	Management discussed and commenced.
15:10	Discharged home.

Clinical presentation

Julia was a second-year nursing student who lived in an apartment with two of her fellow students. She had been studying hard, as well as working 20 hours a week in a part-time job. She had usually been in good health, but recently had been feeling tired and had almost collapsed on two occasions.

This morning she stood up from her desk and promptly fell down, losing consciousness briefly. She was pale and sweaty, but recovered fully within 10 minutes. One of her fellow students drove her to the emergency department to be assessed.

09:53 hours

Julia presents to the triage desk and is briefly assessed by the triage nurse. She was well, with normal vital signs, and was assigned a triage category of 4—ideally to be seen within 60 minutes. She sat down in the waiting room and waited to be taken in to the department.

10:32 hours

Julia was feeling restless sitting in the waiting room and stood up to go for a short walk. As she stood up, she complained of feeling light-headed and called for help. Her friend and the triage nurse caught her as she began to collapse, and together they laid her down. She was lifted from the floor onto a trolley and promptly taken into a cubicle inside the department. She did not lose consciousness on this occasion.

She was greeted by an emergency nurse who commenced an assessment and began taking observations.

The vital signs were recorded as:

- PR   84 bpm
- BP   110/70 lying, 70/30 standing
- RR   16 breaths/minute
- Blood sugar level   6.2 mmol/L

The nurse proceeded to take a 12-lead ECG, which is shown in Figure 1.1 below.

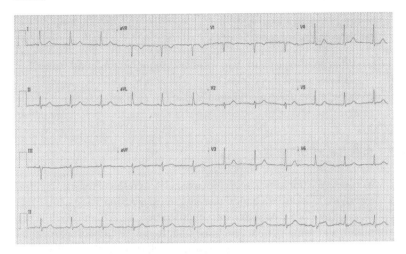

Figure 1.1 ECG

Physiology comment

The determinants of mean arterial pressure are cardiac output (heart rate × stroke volume) and total peripheral resistance. As a person moves from lying down to an upright position, cardiac output tends to fall by approximately 20% because gravity reduces the venous return to the right side of the heart. This fall in cardiac output is partially offset by several autonomically mediated reflexes that act to minimise the fall in cardiac output by simultaneously increasing heart rate, stroke volume and peripheral resistance.

A decreased venous return leads to a fall in the right atrial volume and stretch, which ultimately leads to a drop in stroke volume and a drop in arterial pressure. Baroreceptors quickly sense this drop in pressure and elicit an increased sympathetic output that increases heart rate and contractility and total peripheral resistance (TPR). One or a combination of the following may cause the poor orthostatic response seen in the patient:

- Reduced ability of autonomic nervous system to increase heart rate and stroke volume and therefore cardiac output
- Reduced ability of the autonomic nervous system to increase TPR
- Reduced total blood volume
- Maldistribution of blood volume.

Clinical question 1

(a) What are the possible diagnoses and, with these in mind, how will you assess this patient?
(b) What is the value of a 12-lead ECG in this setting?

Clinical comment

Syncope is the transient loss of consciousness as a result of reduced cerebral perfusion. This case is a typical presentation of syncope. It is essential that the treating doctor consider important causes of such an event. When initially assessing patients such as Julia, it can be helpful to consider what the possible causes could be, and to ask specifically for diagnostic symptoms and to look for signs that may suggest the underlying cause.

Important causes of syncope, with examples, include:

- Cardiac causes: arrhythmias (such as long QT syndrome, or other tachyarrhythmias or bradyarrhythmias), myocardial ischaemia, aortic valve stenosis, or hypertrophic obstructive cardiomyopathy (HOCM)
- Vascular causes: pulmonary embolism
- Hypovolaemia: gastrointestinal bleed, ruptured aortic aneurysm, ruptured ectopic pregnancy, or dehydration
- Neurological: subarachnoid haemorrhage, or transient ischaemic attack (TIA)
- Orthostatic hypotension: endocrine causes (such as diabetes mellitus or Addison's disease), or drugs (such as antihypertensives, diuretics, phenothiazines and nitrates)
- Cough or defaecation syncope
- Neurocardiogenic ('vasovagal') causes.

There are a large number of possible diagnoses, but some of them would be very unlikely in a young patient such as Julia. Your initial history and examination would be directed towards diagnosing or ruling out one of these causes. A 12-lead ECG is an essential bedside investigation in this circumstance, as it can diagnose life-threatening causes of syncope such as arrhythmias and myocardial ischaemia.

10:40 hours

You are working as an intern in the emergency department and 'click on' to Julia. You walk into the cubicle just as the nurse completes recording the ECG and hands it to you. You note that the ECG appears to be normal, and in particular that the QT interval is within normal limits.

You introduce yourself to Julia. She describes feeling light-headed over the past week, and this worsens when she stands up. She has fallen down three times, but does not think that she has lost consciousness. She recovers rapidly once she lies back down.

You learn that she is in good health, with no significant past medical history. She has not suffered from palpitations, diarrhoea and vomiting, and she denies that she could be pregnant. It does not appear that she was incontinent of urine, had a prolonged recovery, or had bitten her tongue, suggesting no seizure activity. She denies headaches, visual disturbances, or recent breathlessness.

In your examination you note that she looks dehydrated: she has dry lips, and her tongue appears coated. There is no audible heart murmur, and her lung fields are clear. You ask again about any symptoms of gastroenteritis and about her fluid intake, but she denies anything abnormal. After a brief pause, she looks at you and mentions that there *is* something else: for the past week she has been taking some of her mother's blood pressure tablets to help with weight loss.

Clinical question 2

(a) Given this information, what is the most likely diagnosis?
(b) What further information do you require and what investigations should be performed?

This information prompts you to ask further questions. She produces the medication, and you discover that it is a thiazide diuretic. You are particularly interested in her electrolyte balance, and whether there are any symptoms and signs of a disturbance of her body image. You measure her height as 170 cm and weight as 61 kg, which establishes that she has a body mass index (BMI) of 21.1.

You now decide to insert an intravenous cannula and collect blood for pathology analysis. You request urea and electrolytes (U&Es) and a full blood count (FBC). You request that a urine dipstick be checked for signs of infection and pregnancy. In this instance you delay commencing any therapy until the blood results are available. You go and see another patient while you wait for the blood results.

Clinical question 3

What blood results do you predict?

Physiology comment

A key role of the kidney is the removal of metabolic wastes from the body. It must be remembered that the kidney is also responsible for several other key functions including regulation of water and electrolyte balance, excretion of drugs, regulation of blood pressure, regulation of red blood cell production, regulation of vitamin D production and gluconeogenesis.

Water and electrolyte balance requires body input and output to match so a constant total body amount is maintained. The input of water and electrolytes varies significantly from day to day, and the kidneys respond by varying the amount of water and different electrolytes in the urine to maintain total body balance. The renal system is the only major pathway that the body is able to regulate to alter output of water and most common electrolytes. Not only is the plasma volume filtered through the kidney several times in one day, but also the healthy kidney is able to regulate excretion of the different ions and organics independently, enabling it to maintain subtle control over total body levels.

Clinical comment

The initial assessment served as a screening test for important causes of syncope, and there was little in the history and examination to suggest a sinister cause such as pulmonary embolism or subarachnoid haemorrhage. The clinical examination revealed up to 5% dehydration, as evidenced by dry mucous membranes, and a significant postural drop in blood pressure, which is consistent with the history that emerged. See Table 1.1 below for a classification of dehydration states. Once a rapport had been established, the patient felt that she could talk freely and mentioned the critical history of taking diuretic medication for weight loss.

Diuretics reduce blood pressure by increasing the renal loss of sodium and water. Side effects of this can be electrolyte disturbances, such as hyponatraemia and hypokalaemia. Clinical signs result mainly from the hypovolaemia, though marked electrolyte disturbances can produce a range of symptoms and signs. In this instance it would be reasonable to investigate further and request targeted pathology tests. As therapy can differ vastly depending upon the hydration state and the electrolyte results, and given that the patient is not immediately compromised, it

Table 1.1 Clinical findings of dehydration

Symptom/sign	Mild dehydration (3–5% of body weight)	Moderate dehydration (6–9% of body weight)	Severe dehydration (>10% of body weight)
Level of consciousness	Alert	Lethargic	Obtunded
Capillary refill	2 seconds	2–4 seconds	Greater than 4 seconds, cool limbs
Mucous membranes	Normal	Dry	Parched, cracked
Tears	Normal	Decreased	Absent
Heart rate	Slight increase	Increased	Very increased
Respiratory rate	Normal	Increased	Increased and hyperpnoea
Blood pressure	Normal	Normal, but orthostasis	Decreased
Pulse	Normal	Thready	Faint or impalpable
Skin turgor	Normal	Slow	Tenting
Eyes	Normal	Sunken	Very sunken
Urine output	Decreased	Oliguria	Oliguria/anuria

Note: 1% = 10 mL/kg of body weight

is reasonable to wait before commencing therapy such as intravenous fluid replacement.

Of course, the issues surrounding weight loss and body image will need to be explored further and referrals made as required.

Physiology comment

The concept of the body fluid compartments and their interrelationships is integral to an understanding of hydration state, and specifically of dehydration. Approximately 60% of a person's total body weight is water. Individual variation is primarily attributable to variation in the percentage of body fat, as adipose tissue contains less water than muscle. The percentage of body weight that can be attributed to water is higher in neonates than in adults, at approximately 75%. Total body water can be subdivided into water that resides outside the cells (extracellular fluid [ECF]; approximately 20% of total body weight), and water residing inside cells (intracellular fluid [ICF]; approximately 40% of total body weight). The extracellular fluid can be further subdivided into the fluid between cells (interstitial fluid; approximately 75% of the extracellular fluid), and the plasma (approximately 25% of extracellular fluid). See below:

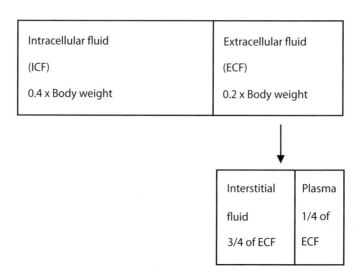

Intracellular fluid	Extracellular fluid
(ICF)	(ECF)
0.4 x Body weight	0.2 x Body weight

Interstitial fluid	Plasma
3/4 of ECF	1/4 of ECF

Physiology comment

All exchange between the body and the external environment occurs through the plasma compartment. For example, fluid and electrolytes lost through diarrhoea comes directly from the plasma compartment because fluid and ions are lost from the splanchnic circulation into the small intestine. Over time, alteration in the volume and composition of the plasma compartment will have an impact on the makeup of the interstitial compartment and, secondarily, the intracellular compartment. To some degree therefore the internal cell environment is buffered from environmental influences, and this helps to maintain a constant homeostatic environment for normal cell function.

The net balance between water input (diet) and output (urinary, GI and evaporative losses) determines the overall total body water (TBW) volume. The division of TBW between the different body water compartments is a function of the amount of solute in each compartment because water can pass freely across the capillary endothelium and cell membrane, driven by any differences in solute concentration between compartments. Most importantly, the volumes of the extracellular compartments depend primarily on the amount of Na and associated anions, since these constitute 90–95% of the total osmotically active ions in the ECF. Factors that deplete total body sodium will therefore be associated with a low ECF volume, while sodium retention is associated with an expanded ECF volume.

Common causes of sodium loss, and therefore hypovolaemia, include:

- GI sodium loss: vomiting, or diarrhoea
- Renal sodium loss: *diuretics*, or tubulointerstitial disease
- Direct loss (haemorrhage)
- Other routes: sweating, or burns.

Common causes of sodium gain and therefore hypervolaemia include primarily the inability of the kidneys to excrete Na at high enough rates to maintain external (input and output) balance. For example, in cases of congestive heart failure the kidney inappropriately reabsorbs Na and water, expanding the ECF volume, and in chronic renal failure the reduction in glomerular filtration rate reduces the kidneys' capacity to excrete Na, leading to hypervolaemia.

Dehydration therefore can be thought of in terms of a deficit in total body water (i.e. a negative balance between input and output), and the term 'hypovolaemia' can be used to describe specifically a deficit in the plasma volume.

12:30 hours

The blood results are available, and are displayed in Table 1.2 below.

Table 1.2 Blood results

Result	Level	Normal range
Na	132	135–145 mmol/L
K	3.4	3.5–4.5 mmol/L
Cl	96	95–110 mmol/L
Urea	5.4	3.0–8.0 mmol/L
Creatinine	0.045	< 0.120 mmol/L
Hb	167	115–165 g/L
WCC	5.8	$4.0–11.0 \times 10^9/L$
Platelets	231	$150–400 \times 10^9/L$

Physiology comment

Diuretics are a group of drugs that increase the urinary excretion of sodium and water by inhibiting the reabsorption of sodium ions by the nephron. The site of inhibition in the nephron varies with each particular type of diuretic. Thiazide diuretics are used more for the treatment of hypertension than for the aggressive reduction of extracellular fluid volume, and this is the context for their initial prescription in this case. These drugs reduce sodium and chloride reabsorption by inhibiting the Na–Cl symporter in the early distal tubule. This leads to a higher solute load in the collecting duct, which opposes fluid reabsorption in this and the following segment, thus producing a diuresis. Thiazide use will therefore increase the renal excretion of sodium and chloride and water, leading to the electrolyte pattern seen in the blood results. Thiazide use also increases renal potassium loss, increasing the potential for lowered plasma potassium levels to develop (hypokalaemia), by the following three mechanisms:

1 The decrease in extracellular volume induced by the diuretic action activates the renin–angiotensin system and thus aldosterone levels. This rise in plasma aldosterone ultimately stimulates potassium secretion from principal cells in the late distal tubule and collecting duct.

2 Increased delivery of sodium to principal cells increases the rate of potassium secretion from the same cells. The increased sodium delivery leads to an increase in the activity of NaKATPase pumps located on the basolateral membrane, driving more potassium into the cell and so enhancing secretion. The reabsorption of sodium also provides a favourable electrical gradient for the movement of potassium in the opposite direction across the luminal membrane.

3 The increased rate of tubular flow stimulates greater potassium secretion from principal cells. This is because the final step for the movement of potassium from the cell into the tubular lumen is passive down its concentration gradient, through a potassium-specific ion channel. A fast flow rate lowers the concentration of potassium on the luminal side of the cell membrane, maximising the concentration gradient across the membrane and leading to a higher rate of movement of potassium out of the cell.

Clinical question 4

Describe the results. How do they assist you with your assessment and management?

Clinical comment

The blood results are consistent with mild dehydration secondary to diuretic use: there is haemoconcentration, with a raised haemoglobin, and sodium, potassium and chloride are mildly reduced. These should revert to normal simply by discontinuing the diuretic and encouraging a normal fluid intake.

Physiology comment

Care must be taken to keep an underlying assessment of hydration status in mind when reviewing electrolyte values. Electrolyte concentration may be elevated even though there is an overall total body deficit of that electrolyte. This is not because total body electrolyte has increased, but because relatively more water than electrolyte has been lost. Care must always be taken, therefore, to interpret electrolyte values along with an assessment of body fluid status.

In this case the diuretic use has caused both a decrease in total body sodium, potassium and chloride, and an overall loss of water. The slightly lowered electrolyte values indicate a picture of significant electrolyte loss with a slightly lower proportional loss of water. Normal fluid intake will quickly restore the lost volume, and the kidney will respond to limit further electrolyte losses, enabling dietary intake to replace the overall total body electrolyte deficit quickly.

12:45 hours

You discuss the results with Julia, and explain the effects of the diuretic use. You establish that this is not a long-term problem—she had been taking the tablets as a 'quick' way of losing weight. Her BMI is within the healthy range, and there is no evidence that she has any problem with her body image. However, you explain that medication can have serious side-effects, and that casual self-medication can be dangerous. She reassures you that she has learned her lesson and will stop using the medication.

She still feels quite faint when she stands up; so you decide to start replacing intravascular volume with one litre of isotonic normal saline (N/S) over two hours, with a view to reassessing her status when the infusion is complete.

15:10 hours

Julia is feeling much better—she no longer feels unwell with postural changes, and her blood pressure remains the same on standing. She is discharged home with advice to stop taking the medication and to maintain a fluid intake of at least 5 glasses of water a day.

Epilogue

Julia stopped taking the diuretics and her symptoms resolved after two days. She was followed up by her GP, who received a discharge letter from the emergency department.

Tips

- Syncope is a common presentation in emergency departments, and simple investigations such as a blood glucose level and an ECG are essential in making a diagnosis.
- A directed clinical examination must include measuring for postural blood pressure changes.
- 0.9% normal saline is a cheap and effective intravenous fluid to use for rehydration.
- Be alert to 'red flag' symptoms and signs of serious underlying conditions, and investigate and manage them appropriately.

Clinical summary

This case presents a diagnostic challenge. Serious conditions have the potential to present in a variety of ways, some obvious but some subtle. Syncope accounts for 1–3% of emergency department presentations, so it is essential that medical staff are able to differentiate serious from benign aetiologies in a timely manner. A number of decision-making aids have been developed and validated, with varying degrees of accuracy. Large-scale studies have identified a number of warning signs, and their presence should mandate admission for observation and further investigation:

1 Abnormal ECG
2 Focal neurological signs
3 Abnormal cardiac signs: the presence of a murmur, for example
4 Any clinical suspicion of a significant cause: such as pulmonary embolism, subarachnoid haemorrhage or ectopic pregnancy.

Definitive management will be determined by the final diagnosis, but as is often the case in emergency practice, some therapy may have to be started while the assessment is being undertaken. Hypotension with signs of shock should be treated aggressively by fluid replacement, and 0.9% normal saline is the most appropriate intravenous fluid to use. A range of fluids are available to use when fluid replacement is required, and there are a number of issues to consider prior to commencing such therapy:

1 Is fluid replacement actually required?
Treating doctors should carefully assess whether such therapy is actually necessary—oral rehydration may well be adequate. Intravenous cannulation can cause complications

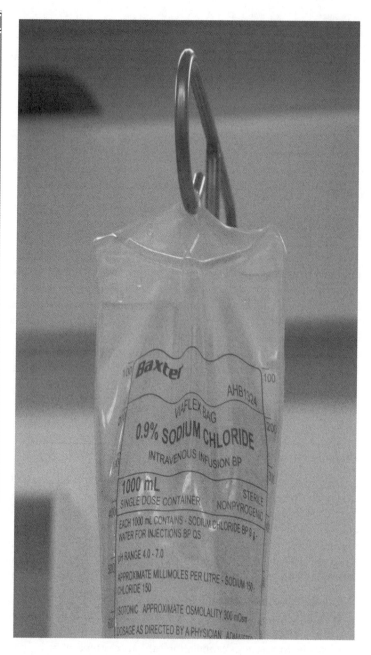

Figure 1.2 One litre bag of normal saline prepared for infusion

such as thrombophlebitis, and excess amounts of fluid may be unintentionally administered, resulting in pulmonary oedema.

2 What fluid should be used?

0.9% sodium chloride, as seen in Figure 1.2 and otherwise referred to as 'normal saline', is a safe, cheap and ubiquitous fluid often used in emergency departments. It is isotonic with plasma; so it will not usually result in electrolyte abnormalities if administered in standard volumes. It is ideal for fluid replacement in dehydration secondary to gastroenteritis, and in the first-line treatment of hypovolaemic shock. Hartmann's, or 'Ringer's lactate', is used for similar purposes but contains potassium and lactate, and is more consistent with plasma values. It is often used in elective surgery and maintenance fluid for inpatients.

Other fluids available include 5% dextrose, which rapidly becomes hypotonic once the dextrose is metabolised. It is often used to administer intravenous medication by infusion, such as glyceryl trinitrate. It should be used if an excess of water is required to be replaced, as would occur in a patient with hypernatraemia caused predominantly by fluid depletion.

3 At what rate should fluid be administered?

Fluid should be administered at a rate that corrects the deficit appropriately. Long-term injury may follow if it is administered too slowly and perfusion is not restored. On the other hand, while the rapid infusion of intravenous fluid may be well tolerated by a dehydrated adolescent, it could precipitate pulmonary oedema in an elderly patient with pre-existing cardiac disease, or cerebral oedema in a child with diabetic ketoacidosis. It must be emphasised that, when treating children, treating clinicians must consider the child's weight and administer fluid based on a millilitre per kilogram of body weight basis (e.g. 10 mL/kg as a bolus and then re-assess).

4 What are the end-points of the therapy?

The short-term aim of administering fluid is to restore intravascular volume and perfusion of end-organs. Assessing the conscious state, peripheral perfusion, urine output and postural blood pressure are useful parameters to consider.

In Julia's case, intravenous fluid replacement was chosen because of her substantial fall in blood pressure with postural changes and because the cause of the syncopal event was certain. The practice of administering a defined volume and then assessing its effect was applied: the patient felt better after one litre of 0.9% normal saline, and hence no further treatment was required.

This case illustrates the application of clinical guidelines and protocols and the need for risk stratification to play a role in clinical decision-making. This important principle will be illustrated in all the cases presented in this book.

References and further reading

1 American College of Emergency Physicians, Clinical policy: Critical issues in the evaluation and management of patients presenting with syncope. *Ann Emerg Med* Jun 2001; 37: 771–6.
2 Brown, A.F.T. & Cadogan, M.D. *Emergency medicine—Emergency and acute medicine: Diagnosis and management*, 5th edn, Hodder Arnold, London, 2007.
3 Ellsbury, D.L. & George, C.S. Dehydration, eMedicine <www.emedicine.com/ped/topic556.htm> accessed 12 Feb 2009.
4 Reed, M.J. & Gray, A. Collapse query cause: The management of adult syncope in the emergency department. *Emerg Med J* 2006; 23: 589–94.
5 Reed, M.J., Newby, D.E., Coull, A.J. et al. The Risk stratification Of Syncope in the Emergency department (ROSE) pilot study: A comparison of existing syncope guidelines. *Emerg Med J* 2007; 24: 270–5.
6 Sun, B.J., Mangione, C.M., Merchant, G. et al. External validation of the San Francisco syncope rule. *Ann Emerg Med* 2007; 49: 420–7.

Case review

Basic science questions

1 The primary mechanism of action of thiazide diuretics is to:
   A Inhibit Na–Cl cotransport in the distal convoluted tubule
   B Block the direct reabsorption of Na in the thick ascending limb of the Loop of Henle
   C Prevent $NaHCO_3$ reabsorption by limiting H formation
   D Directly block apical Na channels
   E Antagonise aldosterone

2 Dehydration is best described as a decrease in:
   A ECF volume
   B ICF volume
   C Total body water
   D Interstitial volume
   E Plasma volume

3 Hypervolaemia is associated with which of the following conditions?
   A Vomiting
   B Diarrhoea
   C Diuretic use

D Haemorrhage

E Chronic renal failure

Clinical questions

1 Match the following symptoms with the most likely cause of syncope.

  A A 45-year-old female collapses after a getting off a 16 hour flight.

  B A 19-year-old female complains of left-sided low abdominal pain and then faints. She looks pale and sweaty.

  C A 79-year-old male complains of palpitations and then feels light headed. When he is assessed he has a normal ECG.

  D A 27-year-old male complains of the sudden onset of a severe headache and faints.

  E A 63-year-old male feels faint and is noted to have slurred speech for approximately 15 minutes, and then recovers fully.

   (i) Subarachnoid haemorrhage

   (ii) Transient ischaemic attack

   (iii) Ectopic pregnancy

   (iv) Pulmonary embolism

   (v) Paroxysmal atrial fibrillation

2 Which of the following patients with syncope could most likely be safely discharged from the emergency department (ED) with minimal investigation and no further follow-up?

  A A 56-year-old male has a short episode of palpitations. He has a normal ECG in the ED and has normal blood results after a period of observation.

  B A 17-year-old female who by dates is 7 weeks pregnant presents with a faint. She is now well.

  C A 32-year-old male with gastroenteritis and who is mildly dehydrated falls over when standing up to urinate. He has now recovered.

  D A 27-year-old male complains of 2 hours of a throbbing headache with visual disturbance and paraesthesia in his left arm.

  E A 63-year-old female collapses without warning and now feels well, with only a mild tachycardia and normal physical examination.

3 When using intravenous fluids to rehydrate a young patient with normal electrolyte balance, which would be the most appropriate fluid to use?

  A 5% dextrose

  B 0.9% NaCl ('normal saline')

  C 4% dextrose / 0.18% NaCl ('four-and-a-fifth')

  D A colloid, such as Haemaccel

  E 1.8% NaCl ('twice normal saline')

Case 2
Ailsa was feeling the heat …

It's a scorcher of a day, with the town in the middle of a week-long heatwave. The emergency department is preparing for an influx of patients, but as an intern you're not sure what to expect. You try to keep an open mind as you log on to your next patient, a usually well 77-year-old woman named Ailsa.

Clinical learning objectives

- Describe your approach to the patient who presents with a fall and a resulting injury.
- Be able to classify and diagnose heat-related illnesses.
- Be able to assess a patient's hydration status and begin appropriate fluid therapy.
- Understand the complications that can arise from significant dehydration.
- Learn how to use and interpret pathology tests appropriately in the assessment of a patient presenting with syncope.

Physiology learning objectives

- Identify which plasma components can be used as markers for renal function.
- Define hypernatraemia and review its various physiological causes.
- Describe how sodium balance is regulated.
- Discuss how evaluation of extracellular volume can indicate the physiological cause of hypernatraemia.
- Describe the causes and consequences of a metabolic acidosis.
- Discuss renal and respiratory compensation in metabolic acidosis.

Timeline

11:35	Ailsa falls at home, remains on floor.
13:55	Reaches phone, calls for an ambulance.
14:40	Ambulance arrives, transports her to hospital.
15:10	Arrival at hospital; triaged category 3 as 'fall, injured left hip'; nurse initiates analgesia.
15:55	Seen by medical staff and assessment begins.
17:35	Initial results available and directed management starts.
17:50	ABG taken, referrals made.
22.30	Bed available on ward.

Clinical presentation

Ailsa was a spritely 77-year-old woman who had lived alone independently for the 5 years since her husband died. She had hypertension, and apart from osteoarthritis in her knees she was in good health. The summer had been warm, and the past few days had seen the temperature consistently at 8–10° Celsius above the average. She had tried to cope with the heat, but was finding it increasingly hard to get around to perform her usual activities—everything was so hot, and she was feeling breathless and weak. Electricity rationing and power failures had made life even more uncomfortable as she was unable to run her ceiling fan.

Walking from the kitchen to the lounge room, she felt particularly unwell and collapsed to the floor. Coming to, what she thought was only a few seconds later, she became aware of a pain in her left hip, and she was unable to rise. She crawled slowly to the telephone, and called for an ambulance. Being particularly stoic, she reported only that she had fallen and injured her hip and couldn't get up. To the ambulance dispatcher this did not sound particularly urgent, and so the next available non-urgent crew was dispatched. As most of the city's ambulances were 'ramped', waiting to off-load patients into the emergency department, this took longer than usual. Once the crew arrived they removed her promptly from her house and transported her to the local hospital. After being triaged Ailsa was offered analgesia for her painful hip, and transferred to a bed in a cubicle. A member of the nursing staff began his assessment; to hasten the assessment he inserted an intravenous cannula and collected a series of blood samples.

15:55 hours

It's been a busy day for the junior staff in the department. The number of patients through has been above the average, dominated by those most vulnerable during such an extreme environmental event—the young and the elderly. You have just started work for the 16:00–01:00 shift, and log on to see Ailsa. The triage notes describe her as 'fall, injured left hip', and you expect that this should be a fairly straight-forward patient. You enter the cubicle and introduce yourself to Ailsa.

You quickly learn that she looks after herself well, and that she has not been in a hospital for many years. Ailsa describes pain in her left hip, which is worse on movement. She does not appear to have suffered any other injuries, and denies hitting her head. Her vital signs are as follows:

- PR   110 bpm
- BP   105/50
- RR   20
- Temperature   38.6°C

Her skin is dry and her lips and tongue are thick and coated, not at all moist. Her eyes appear sunken. Other clinical examination is otherwise unremarkable, apart from localised tenderness to her left hip region.

Clinical question 1

(a) What is your initial impression?
(b) What issues must be considered in a patient such as Ailsa in this situation?
(c) What are your provisional diagnoses?

Clinical comment

It would be a grave error to consider Ailsa's painful left hip in isolation. While it may be tempting to think of her as suffering only a fractured neck of femur, a more detailed history must be sought. Issues such as the cause for the fall, her social situation, her overall falls' risk and predisposition to falls must be considered. As discussed in Case 1, the clinician must be able to recognise syncope as a cause for a fall or any other presenting symptoms. Important causes of syncope were covered in Case 1. In this instance, the patient appears to be significantly dehydrated, with up to 6–9% of her body water lost. If her body weight is 60 kg, this represents a deficit of around 4–5 L of body fluids, and this must be replaced carefully. Replacement that is too rapid can lead to complications, such as pulmonary oedema and more electrolyte disturbances, especially in the elderly. Strict fluid balance is essential. Monitoring urine output using an indwelling catheter is the best way to assess the patient's response to therapy.

Longer term management issues should be considered. Many emergency departments have multidisciplinary aged care teams that can assess living arrangements, conduct risk assessments, and recommend home-based interventions. The use of such teams exemplifies the value of interprofessional training—few doctors have the skills necessary to access such knowledge and resources, yet they must know about referral patterns and other available skills.

Additionally, early pain relief is of paramount importance—intravenous access should be obtained early and opioid analgesia titrated to relieve pain. Effective regional anaesthesia, such as a femoral nerve or a '3 in 1' block, can provide effective long-acting pain relief without the side-effects of repeated parenteral analgesia.

Your working diagnosis is dehydration and heat exhaustion leading to a fall that resulted in a fractured left neck of femur.

You become aware that Ailsa is in pain, and that the pain is likely to get worse when she is moved about the department and transferred for X-rays. The nurse has obtained intravenous access and collected blood; you provide intravenous morphine in 2.5 mg increments. Under supervision from the registrar, you perform a femoral nerve block with 15 mL of 0.25% bupivicaine and 5 mL of 1% lignocaine, which provides rapid relief. You arrange X-rays and begin intravenous rehydration with 0.9% normal saline infused at the rate of 1 L over 4 hours. An indwelling catheter is passed, for the patient's comfort while she has a painful left hip and for the more important and acute reason of monitoring fluid balance. Noting the hot day outside and Ailsa's temperature of 38.6°, you remove her clothing except for a gown, and arrange for a fan to be placed next to her to blow cool air over her body in an attempt to cool her.

Aware of the lack of inpatient beds at the hospital, you place an admission request for a bed for Ailsa in the orthopaedic unit. This is commonly done as early as possible to streamline admission and improve patient flow—the fact is, Ailsa can't go home today whether there's a fracture or not, or whether her blood tests are normal or not. The decision to admit has already been made. You do wonder if a higher level of care might be necessary in the first 24 hours, however, and plan to call the high dependency unit for a review. You present your assessment and plan to the consultant emergency physician, who reviews the patient with you and agrees with your actions so far.

Clinical question 2

What blood tests and X-rays and other investigations would you request, and what results would you be expecting? Justify your answers.

Clinical comment

The two immediate issues to consider are the cause of the fall and the consequences of the fall. In order to address these issues logically and effectively it is useful to think of them as discrete events, each with its own assessment and management requirements.

As discussed in Case 1, syncope is a common cause of presentations to emergency departments. In this instance, an ECG should be performed to look for signs of arrhythmia, ischaemia, or electrolyte abnormality. A blood glucose level can also be performed easily at the bedside, and can identify hypoglycaemia, an important but easily treatable cause of collapse. You have already made the clinical assessment that Ailsa is dehydrated; so investigations should be directed towards assessing the consequences of the dehydration.

Specific blood tests could include:

- Full blood count: looking for signs of anaemia, but also haemoconcentration
- Urea and electrolytes: some renal dysfunction could be expected, as would disturbances in sodium, potassium and calcium
- Creatinine kinase: this could be elevated due to rhabdomyolysis, but is not requested when looking for myocardial damage unless the ECG and history suggest it as a possible cause
- Coagulation profile and blood group and hold: with a view to requiring an operation to internally fixate a likely fractured hip.

Specific X-rays would include pelvis and left hip and a chest X-ray (again, performed as part of a pre-operative work-up). Other imaging would be performed only if clinically indicated—for example, a CT scan of her brain if there was evidence of a head injury, and other X-rays once a secondary survey had been performed to look for other injuries.

17:35 hours

The results are back (see Table 2.1 below); you have been busy seeing two other patients in the meantime. It's your third week in the emergency department and your time management skills are improving significantly. Ailsa remains comfortable—the femoral nerve block seems to have worked quite well. Her temperature has reduced to 37°C. The 12-lead ECG by the bedside shows no acute changes consistent with ischaemia or an electrolyte disturbance, and the finger-prick blood glucose is 6.4 mmol/L.

Table 2.1 Blood test results

Result	Level	Normal range
Na	152	135–145 mmol/L
K	5.4	3.5–4.5 mmol/L
Cl	110	95–110 mmol/L
HCO_3	16	22–32 mmol/L
Urea	13.2	3.0–8.0 mmol/L
Creatinine	0.193	< 0.120 mmol/L
CK	11450	< 200 mmol/L
Hb	190	115–165 g/L
WCC	5.8	$4.0–11.0 \times 10^9$/L
Platelets	231	$150–400 \times 10^9$/L

The X-rays are available, and are shown in Figure 2.1 below:

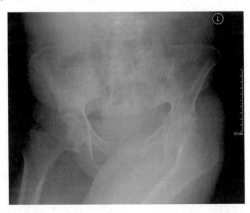

Figure 2.1 X-ray of pelvis

Clinical question 3

Interpret the results and describe your management plan.

Physiology comment

Plasma creatinine as a marker of renal function

Creatine phosphate is a limited-capacity intracellular energy store that is quickly accessed, and when it is broken down it releases creatinine. This release of creatinine into the plasma is relatively constant and is proportional to an individual's muscle mass. Temporary increases in input and therefore plasma concentration do occur after intensive exercise or certain high-protein meals, but generally speaking an elevation in plasma concentration can be attributed to decreased loss from the plasma. As the renal system is the only major pathway for elimination of creatinine in the body, decreased output is caused by either a temporary or permanent impairment of renal function. As renal function and therefore the glomerular filtration rate falls, the elimination of creatinine is reduced and creatinine builds up in the body. As excretion depends on both the plasma concentration and the glomerular filtration rate, the plasma concentration does not continue to rise unchecked: it rises only to the point at which the decrease in GFR is offset by the rise in plasma concentration and a new steady-state equilibrium is established. If the plasma concentration of creatinine can be measured by blood sampling and the input can be estimated (from body weight), a relatively accurate assessment of GFR can be obtained, with a lower GFR associated with higher plasma creatinine levels. As plasma creatinine rises exponentially as GFR drops, the estimate of GFR from plasma creatinine becomes more accurate the lower the GFR becomes. The practical implication is that mild renal insufficiency cannot be reliably assessed using plasma creatinine, but more severe renal dysfunction can be usefully investigated and tracked using plasma creatinine.

In Ailsa's case, the reduced circulating volume has caused a reflex reduction in GFR. This reduced GFR has caused an imbalance in creatinine input and output, leading to a new elevated steady-state creatinine concentration being established. A creatinine of 0.193 mmol/L equates to a GFR of 23 mL/min/1.73 m², a low value that indicates very poor renal functionality, primarily caused by underperfusion of the kidneys.

Physiology comment

Hypernatraemia can be defined as a plasma sodium concentration greater than 145 mmol/L. It can be caused by either a relative increase in total body sodium relative to body water or a relative deficit in body water relative to total body sodium.

Given the two possible causes of hypernatraemia it is important to have a good understanding of how body water (see physiology comment on pp 8–9) and total body sodium levels are regulated. For both sodium and water, a constant body volume or amount is reliant on an equilibrium between input and output. As long as input is equal to output then total body amounts/volumes will not change. An imbalance in either factor or both can lead to the development of hypernatraemia.

Sodium balance

Intake or input of sodium into the body is through dietary intake, with a typical Western diet often including upwards of 10 g of sodium per day. Unlike water intake, which is regulated by the thirst response, sodium intake does not seem to be regulated directly, with intake being primarily related to habit and availability. The unregulated loss (*output*) of Na is primarily through the GI tract and skin, and the amounts lost through these pathways are typically much smaller than the amount taken in, at around 0.5 g per day. The renal system is therefore required to excrete the balance of approximately 9.5 g on a daily basis to maintain a constant total body sodium amount.

Input Na		Output Na
Dietary intake of 6–12 g per day	For steady state input = output	Renal excretion regulated through GFR, amount reabsorbed (aldosterone)

Renal sodium excretion is regulated by variation in both the glomerular filtration rate and the amount of sodium reabsorbed, primarily in the latter part of the nephron. If total body sodium is elevated, GFR is reflexly increased and sodium reabsorbtion in the nephron reduced, leading to increased output. The opposite occurs when total body sodium is reduced. Plasma sodium concentration does not influence GFR and sodium reabsorption directly; instead both are influenced indirectly by the effect of elevated total body sodium levels on blood volume and therefore blood pressure.

The elevated blood pressure associated with a high total body sodium increases GFR either directly or via a baroreceptor-mediated sympathetic response. The increased blood pressure also triggers a reduction of sodium reabsorption in the nephron as the renin–angiotensin system (RAAS) becomes inactivated. Reduced activation of the RAAS leads to lowered circulating aldosterone levels, and this is the primary factor that promotes renal sodium excretion. When total body sodium and therefore ECF volume is significantly elevated, a third factor—atrial natriuretic factor or peptide (ANF)—promotes sodium excretion, acting to regulate an upper plasma volume limit. Atrial natriuretic factory or peptide is released from the atria in response to increased stretch, and it increases sodium excretion by influencing both GFR and sodium reabsorption simultaneously.

Evaluation of extracellular volume indicates the physiological cause of any hypernatraemia.

- A hypovolaemic state indicates that there is significant depletion of the extracellular fluid compartment (ECF) as well as coexistent hyper-natraemia. This hypovolaemic state is most likely to have been caused by vomiting or diarrhoea and the simultaneous loss of both fluid and electrolytes. This is the scenario most likely to decrease ECF volume, as minimal secondary shifts from the intracellular fluid compartment (ICF) occur and the volume is almost totally lost from the ECF.
- A near euvolaemic state indicates that the hypernatraemia is likely to have been caused by loss of pure water, which can be caused by inadequate water intake or fever, and results in an initial loss from the ECF. This is quickly compensated for by a secondary shift from the ICF compartment, minimising any change in ECF volume. Hypovolaemic shock is therefore unlikely unless the water loss is extensive.
- A hypervolaemic state indicates that the hypernatraemia is caused by a gain of sodium and associated anions by the body. The gain of sodium can be caused directly by pathways such as isotonic saline infusion, or indirectly through an inability to excrete sodium lead-ing to consequential sodium retention.

Ailsa is suffering from hypernatraemia and coexisting hypovolaemia. The elevated temperature she has experienced during the past several days would have increased fluid loss through sweating, which, combined with a reduced thirst response often seen in the elderly, has led to a significant reduction in her circulating plasma volume and contributed to her weakness and breathlessness.

Clinical comment

The X-rays reveal a fractured subcapital neck of her left femur, which will require operative repair.

The blood tests reveal significant disturbances in Ailsa's physiology. She has moderate acute renal failure and an accompanying hypernatraemia and hyperchloraemia. A low bicarbonate suggests that she has a metabolic acidosis that is most probably a lactic acidosis resulting from the combination of reduced tissue perfusion and the renal dysfunction. The elevated CK confirms rhabdomyolysis, which will further damage Ailsa's renal function and contribute to hyperkalaemia. The elevated haemoglobin suggests significant haemoconcentration, a feature of significant dehydration. These features suggest that Ailsa is suffering from heat stroke (refer to Table 2.2 below).

Fortunately, in the absence of any acute ECG changes, most of these disturbances will correct themselves over the coming days provided fluid management is prudent and she is closely monitored. She is also

Table 2.2 Classification and features of heat-related illnesses. Adapted from Wexler (2002).

Heat cramps	Heat exhaustion	Heatstroke
Elevated body temperature	*Same as heat cramps, plus:*	*Same as heat exhaustion, plus:*
Thirst	Nausea/vomiting	Anhydrosis
Muscle cramps	Headache	Delirium/seizure/coma
Sweating	Malaise/myalgias	Renal failure
Tachycardia	Hypotension	Hepatocellular necrosis
	Lightheadedness/syncope	Hyperventilation
	Oliguria	Pulmonary oedema
	Uncoordination	Arrhythmia
	Confusion	Rhabdomyolysis
	Irritability	Shock

at a greater risk of venous thromboembolism; so in keeping with hospital guidelines prophylactic anticoagulation with 40 U of subcutaneous enoxaparin daily is started. The cornerstone of therapy in this instance remains intravenous rehydration to restore perfusion while being vigilant for further complications.

Ailsa is, of course, not fit for any operative intervention until her electrolytes, renal function and dehydration are corrected.

Given these results, and noting that her chest X-ray (not shown) does not reveal any signs of heart failure, you increase the rate of fluids as shown in Table 2.3 below.

Table 2.3 Fluid Orders

Fluid	Amount	Additives	Rate	Signed
N/S (normal saline)	1000 mL	–	1000 mL/hour	Geoff Couser
N/S	1000 mL	–	500 mL/hour	Geoff Couser
N/S	1000 mL	–	250 mL/hour	Geoff Couser

You observe her closely and reassess her frequently to ensure that these fluids are not administered too quickly for her to manage. Needing to assess her acid–base balance better, and expecting it to reveal significant abnormalities, you take an arterial blood gas. This reveals the results in Table 2.4 below.

Table 2.4 Arterial blood gas results

Result	Level	Normal range
FIO2: 0.21		
pH	7.16	7.35–7.45
pCO2	16	35–45 mmHg
pO2	89	80–100 mmHg
HCO3	14	22–32 mmol/L
Base excess	–9.3	–3 – +3
Blood glucose	6.4	<7.7 mmol/L
Lactate	7.1	<0.8 mmol/L

Clinical question 4

Interpret the ABG. Is it what you were expecting?

Clinical comment

The ABG reveals a partially compensated metabolic acidosis. This is revealed by the low bicarbonate, the low pCO_2 and the low pH. The lactate is elevated, which is consistent with her poorly perfused shocked state. Common causes of a lactic acidosis include:

- Type A: poor perfusion (cardiac arrest, exercise, dehydration, and hypovolaemic shock)
- Type B: (1) medical conditions; (2) drugs; (3) congenital.

The arterial blood gas results are expected, as Ailsa is shocked: she is dehydrated to the point that she has poor perfusion of her end organs, with evidence of end-organ failure. The added load of myoglobin exacerbates the renal dysfunction, which in turn exacerbates the metabolic acidosis.

Physiology comment

Metabolic acidosis is caused by the accumulation of non-volatile acid within the body. There are three important processes that act to limit the impact that the accumulation of acid has on plasma pH: buffering, changes in respiration, and excretion of hydrogen ion by the renal system.

The first of these processes is the buffering of hydrogen by bases, of which the most important is bicarbonate. The free hydrogen ion combines with any available base, effectively removing the hydrogen ion from solution and locking it up in an inactive form. The hydrogen ion still has to be excreted from the body at a later stage, and this occurs through the renal system. Buffering therefore leads to a rapid (within minutes) drop in plasma bicarbonate that is proportional to the degree of acid excess. Other bases also contribute to the body's ability to buffer hydrogen ion, including extracellular and intracellular proteins and a limited amount of phosphate.

During an acidosis the pH will still drop to some degree, even though the bicarbonate buffer system limits the accumulation of free hydrogen ion. This drop in pH acts as potent stimulator to the respiratory system, and the rate and depth of ventilation increase significantly. At the extreme, this breathing pattern (known as Kussmaul's respiration or Kussmaul's breathing), is typified by a very deep gasping type of respiration associated with severe acidosis. Once established, this respiratory pattern very rapidly (within 10s of minutes) drives the $paCO_2$ below the normal 40 mmHg, thus bringing the pH closer to 7.4. This occurs because the carbonic acid equilibrium is driven to the left, reducing the amount of free H^+.

$$\downarrow CO_2 + H_2O \Leftrightarrow H_2CO_3 \Leftrightarrow HCO_3^- + \downarrow H^+$$

This change in ventilatory pattern compensates for the metabolic acidosis and will act to normalise the pH. Even though the pH will approach 7.40, respiratory compensation will never be able to correct the acidosis fully.

Long-term correction of the acidosis requires the kidney to excrete the excess hydrogen ion (or acid load) from the body. This involves different segments of the nephron being stimulated simultaneously to excrete hydrogen ion and add bicarbonate to the peritubular capillaries. In the proximal tubule all filtered bicarbonate is reabsorbed and hydrogen ion secreted; later on down the tubule any additional filtered buffers combine with hydrogen ion, enabling bicarbonate to be added to the plasma. After all the filtered buffer has been depleted, the tubular cells are able to synthesise their own in the form of ammonia. The ammonia combines with secreted hydrogen ion to form ammonium, which is excreted in the urine. The urine pH falls to around 4.5, and the plasma bicarbonate, lowered initially as part of the buffer response, is elevated back up within the normal range. In effect the role of the kidney in compensating for an acidosis can be viewed in two ways:

1 Elimination of the acid load from the body and balancing the additional input of acid with increased output
2 Elevation of plasma bicarbonate to a level that brings the ratio of plasma bicarbonate to carbon dioxide back within the normal range.

The ratio of $[HCO_3]$ to $[0.03pCO_2]$ is 20 : 1 at a neutral pH of 7.4. During an acidosis the ratio typically falls and during an alkalosis the ratio rises. The process of compensation aims to normalise the bicarbonate pCO_2 ratio and therefore the pH by altering plasma bicarbonate levels via the kidney and/or pCO_2 levels via the lungs.

An expected pattern therefore follows from the processes that act to limit the impact of the accumulation of acid on plasma pH. The plasma bicarbonate will initially fall very rapidly, with the magnitude of the initial drop related to the amount and rate of acid accumulation. This is then followed over a matter of minutes to hours by a drop in $paCO_2$, with the impact on ventilation being proportional to the severity of the acidosis and the capacity of the patient to alter ventilation. Finally, over a matter of days, the amount of acid excreted by the kidney will increase, followed by a raising of the plasma HCO_3 back towards normal.

Ailsa has experienced a metabolic acidosis caused by poor perfusion and the accumulation of lactate. The pattern in the ABG indicates that buffering has occurred (low HCO_3) and some respiratory compensation is present (low pCO_2). However, there has not been full renal compensation as the pH is still below normal and the HCO_3 is still depressed. This may be because her kidneys are unable to increase the elimination of hydrogen ion and reabsorb bicarbonate (due to renal impairment), or simply that not enough time has elapsed for full renal compensation to occur.

Realising that Ailsa is ill and will need close monitoring in the short term, you call the intensive care unit to request that she be admitted there until her acute disturbances settle and she is fit for an operation. The orthopaedic registrar is contacted but informed that Ailsa is too ill for immediate treatment. The registrar seems happy with that, as there are six patients awaiting surgery on the ward anyway.

22:30 hours

The fluid therapy continues as a bed is made available in the high dependency unit (HDU). Ailsa is finally transferred there late at night to continue her rehydration and monitoring. The femoral nerve block continues to provide excellent anaesthesia. You note that the urine bag is starting to fill as she is transferred—a sure sign that her kidneys are starting to function properly again.

Clinical comment

This case demonstrates the multifactorial issues that arise in assessing and managing such a patient. Failure to consider the cause of falls and address disturbances in the underlying physiology can lead to significant diagnoses being missed, thus leading to increasing morbidity and mortality.

A fractured neck of femur is a common diagnosis in patients over the age of 70, with a marked increase in incidence with increasing age. It is in the top 20 reasons for hospital admissions in Australia. An important public health priority is the identification of patients at risk of falls and the implementation of strategies to prevent falls. Assessing patients who present with falls, as well as identifying patients at risk of falling, is an important role of staff working in emergency departments. A number of resources have been developed to assist staff to perform such assessments, and these should be used where indicated. A coordinated interdisciplinary approach is essential for these patients to be managed optimally.

Epilogue

Ailsa remained in the HDU for a further 36 hours, receiving intravenous fluid and frequent blood sampling. Her renal function improved steadily and her creatinine kinase declined steadily. By day 3 she was feeling much better, and with her physiology returning to equilibrium she was taken to the operating theatre for the internal fixation of her fracture. She recovered well and was transferred to the rehabilitation unit 10 days post-operatively. She was discharged home once she was mobilising safely and after the occupational therapist had performed a home visit and introduced some modifications, such as handrails in the bathroom and on the front stairs.

Tips

- Over-resuscitation can be as dangerous as under-resuscitation, especially in the elderly. Be careful not to infuse intravenous fluids too rapidly.
- Be guided by pulse rate, peripheral perfusion and urine output when writing further fluid orders, and monitor electrolytes closely.
- Providing effective analgesia quickly is essential when patients present in pain.

References and further reading

1 Australian Institute of Health and Welfare. Australian hospital statistics 2006–07, Health services series no. 31, Cat. no. HSE 55, AIHW, Canberra 2008, p. 205.
2 Boufous, S., Finch, C.F. & Lord, S.R. Incidence of hip fracture in New South Wales: Are our efforts having an effect? *MJA* 2004; 180: 623–6.
3 Knowlton, K., Rotkin-Ellman, M., King, G. et al. The 2006 California heat wave: Impacts on hospitalizations and emergency department visits. *Environ Health Perspect* Jan 2009; 117 (1): 61–7.
4 Pioli, G., Giusti, A. & Barone, A. Orthogeriatric care for the elderly with hip fractures: Where are we? *Aging Clin Exp Res* Apr 2008; 20 (2): 113–22.
5 Wexler, R.K. Evaluation and treatment of heat-related illnesses. *Am Fam Physician* 2002; 65 (11): 2307–14.

Case review

Basic science questions

1 An elevated plasma creatinine level is most likely to be caused by:
   A Impaired renal function
   B Decreased dietary intake of creatinine
   C A low protein diet
   D Excess intake of free water
   E Increased loss of creatinine through the renal system

2 Renal sodium excretion is *regulated* by variation in which two physiological variables?
   A GFR, and dietary sodium intake
   B Gastrointestinal loss, and sweat rate
   C GFR, and sodium excretion
   D Sweat rate, and GFR
   E Gastrointestinal loss, and dietary sodium intake

3 For a pH of 7.4 the ratio of $[HCO_3]$: $[0.03\ pCO_2]$ is:
   A 1 : 1
   B 2 : 1
   C 4 : 1
   D 20 : 1
   E 100 : 1

Clinical questions

1 Match the following clinical features with the approximate degree of dehydration.
   A A bushwalker is hot and sweaty and feels thirsty.
   B An elderly male is found on a hot day with a reduced level of consciousness, a pulse of 130, a BP of 80/50, and has cracked lips and tongue.
   C A 6-month-old baby has 3 days of vomiting and diarrhoea and has a sunken fontanelle, sunken eyes and dry skin, but is looking around the room and has a capillary refill time of 2 seconds.
   D A 37-year-old diabetic woman is thirsty but alert, has polyuria, a raised respiratory rate, and a capillary refill time of 3 seconds.
      (i)   < 3%
      (ii) 6%
      (iii) 9%
      (iv) > 10%

2 Which of the following fluids would be most appropriate to use to rehydrate a patient with significant dehydration?
 A 0.9% normal saline
 B 3% saline
 C A colloid solution, such as Haemaccel
 D 5% dextrose solution

3 A patient comes in sweaty and confused on a hot day where the temperature is above 28°. His breathing is rapid and his pulse is thready and weak. The condition that best describes this scenario is:
 A Heat stroke
 B Heat exhaustion
 C Heat cramps
 D Heat stress

Case 3
Jack couldn't stop vomiting ...

Jack presents with 2 days of vomiting and is now feeling very thirsty. Also, his abdominal pain is getting worse. He calls an ambulance and he's brought to the emergency department looking simply terrible.

Clinical learning objectives

- Describe the various causes of abdominal pain and how they can be differentiated.
- Know the appropriate use of pathology and radiological investigations in the assessment of abdominal pain.
- Describe the initial management that can be implemented in the emergency department regardless of what the final diagnosis is.
- Describe the important clinical issues to consider concerning the fluid management of patients with abdominal pain.

Physiology learning objectives

- Describe the volume and composition of fluid entering the digestive tract.
- Outline the reasons why venous blood that is leaving an actively secreting stomach is alkaline.
- Describe how and why prepyloric and postpyloric vomiting may alter electrolyte and acid–base balance.

Timeline

13:40	Ambulance arrives with Jack at emergency department; triaged as 'abdo pain, vomiting' and assigned triage category 3.
13:52	Nursing assessment begins; consultant in charge makes initial basic assessment and commences initial management.
14:07	Intern starts to see patient, taking history and performing examination.
14:30	Provisional diagnosis considered, investigations requested; assessment and management plan presented to consultant.
15:45	Initial results available and diagnosis confirmed; referral to inpatient team made and inpatient bed sought.
17:30	Jack is transferred to an inpatient bed.

Clinical presentation

Jack is a stoic 84-year-old war veteran who manages to look after himself well and live independently, despite a range of medical problems including an aortic aneurysm repair five years ago. He's lived alone since his wife died of cancer three years ago, and is adamant that he's doing fine. Every now and then he gets some pain in his abdomen associated with bloating and vomiting, but it usually settles down quickly. This time, though, he's not so sure: he hasn't been able to keep anything down for nearly 2 days, his abdomen feels sore all over, and he feels sick. Not wanting to bother anyone and feeling too ill to drive himself to the local hospital, he calls an ambulance. The ambulance crew cannulates him, provides intravenous analgesia, and commences an infusion of Hartmann's solution. He arrives at the hospital 30 minutes later.

13:40 hours

Jack arrives at the hospital feeling a little better after 5 mg of intravenous morphine and 500 mL of IV fluid. The triage nurse assesses him and directs him to a cubicle with a triage category 3 and a description of 'abdo pain and vomiting ?cause'.

13:52 hours

The nurse allocated to the cubicle enters and begins her assessment. She looks at Jack and realises that he is still in pain. The consultant on duty rapidly assesses him and writes up further intravenous analgesia and maintenance fluids. Both nurse and senior doctor have their suspicions as to what the diagnosis could be, and know what needs to be done. Unfortunately for both Jack and the departmental flow, other more pressing matters arise (such as the two chest pain patients and the road trauma patient, who arrive simultaneously); so Jack, while comfortable, will need to wait a little longer until a junior member of staff can conduct a more thorough assessment.

Clinical question 1

(a) What are the system issues present that act to prolong the time to Jack's care in the department?

(b) What changes could be introduced to the system at this point to improve patient flow through this department and hasten Jack's diagnosis and management?

Clinical comment

Even though the junior doctor is yet to even speak to the patient or begin an examination, much has already been done in the assessment and management of this patient. This illustrates the team approach to patient care that does and should occur in emergency departments. Analgesia has been provided and fluid resuscitation has begun. Patient flow is essential in emergency departments, as even small disruptions and delays can have an adverse impact all along the patient-care pathway: ambulances are unable to off-load patients; patients sit in waiting rooms unable to access a treatment area; patients who have been assessed and admitted sit in the emergency department waiting for an inpatient bed to be allocated. These are the features of access block, and much has been done to understand its causes and solutions. It is therefore essential for all staff to understand the processes of the health system as a whole and to work collaboratively towards improving the care of the patient. It is essential to define roles and allocate tasks appropriate to the level of training: consultant staff oversee the whole department and initiate patient care; junior staff work under their direction and supervision; nursing staff can initiate therapy and make generalised decisions about care. The key is that they all work together as a team and respect and understand each other's abilities.

A number of interventions can be introduced to improve patient flow:

1 Streaming similar patients together and harnessing similar processes (known as 'lean thinking')
2 Working with inpatient units to facilitate review and admission
3 Introducing emergency short-stay units and medical assessment and procedure units (two separate but related entities)
4 Appropriate use of staff skills, such as the use of nursing staff to perform procedures while avoiding performing unnecessary repetitive documentation and tasks.

Consultant emergency physicians, while generally keen to allow junior staff the opportunity to assess patients and enhance their learning experience, need to balance these needs with the needs of the patient and the broader needs of the department.

14:07 hours

As the intern on for the shift, you've been seeing your share of patients, but the registrars and consultants seem more interested in the acute myocardial infarction and the patient with multiple injuries from a motor vehicle crash. You click on to Jack's name on the emergency department information system computer and enter the cubicle.

You find a comfortable but ill-looking elderly male who tries to put on a brave face but is obviously in pain and is unwell. You note that some of the work has already been done, as you refer to the note attached to the patient's record:

'2 days of vomiting and abdominal pain
Actions: IV access, 1L N/S over 2 hours, bloods collected, analgesia provided with 2.5 mg increments of intravenous morphine.'

He has received 7.5 mg of morphine so far, and you see a collection of labelled bloods beside the patient. You note from the end of the bed that his mucous membranes are dry and that his abdomen appears distended. The vital signs are recorded:

- PR   124 bpm
- RR   20
- BP   100/55
- Temp   35.8°C
- SpO_2 96% on 8 L O_2/minute

Clinical question 2

(a) What are your initial impressions of Jack?

(b) Which elements of the history and examination must be considered when assessing patients with abdominal pain?

Clinical comment

Jack appears unwell, so it is essential to act in a timely manner. As with most emergency patients, 'assessment and management occur in parallel'. A bowel obstruction seems to be a likely diagnosis based on the information so far, but this does not negate the need for a more thorough assessment, as other possibilities exist.

Abdominal pain accounts for up to 10% of all emergency department presentations, so a logical approach to its assessment is essential. Elderly patients are disproportionately represented in this figure, and have specific diagnostic and management challenges. It is also essential to use investigations such as pathology and radiology appropriately to avoid unnecessary delays in diagnosis and unnecessary costs.

Some examples of features of the history and the examination and their likely related diagnoses are detailed in Table 3.1 overleaf. Once you have made a provisional diagnosis, you will need to perform more assessment to determine further investigation, management and disposition. [Hint: Attempt to consider the diagnosis before uncovering the answer.]

The intern proceeds to take a history from Jack and records the following information in the medical record:

84 yo male; widowed, lives alone independently

Hx: IHD–occasional angina   Meds: Aspirin 100 mg daily
      Cholecystectomy 1975   GTN 0.4 mg S/L prn
      AAA repair (elective) 2004

Presents with 2/7 of abdominal pain and bloating

Crampy, central, no radiation

Vomiting—bile-stained, up to 7–8 times per day

BNO × 2/7, no flatus

No oral intake tolerated

Pain worsened today, called ambulance and presents for R/V

Physical examination reveals a distended abdomen with hyperesonance to percussion, with minimal bowel sounds and peri-umbilical tenderness.

There were no signs of peritonism. No organomegaly was felt, and there were no stigmata of chronic liver disease. Rectal examination revealed an empty rectum with no palpable masses.

Table 3.1 Types of abdominal pain and possible diagnoses

Prominent features of the history or the examination	Possible diagnosis
Colicky right upper quadrant pain with nausea	Biliary colic
Epigastric pain and tenderness	Pancreatitis
Sudden onset of peri-umbilical pain with hypotension in an elderly patient	Ruptured aortic aneurysm
Peri-umbilical pain moving to the right iliac fossa associated with guarding	Appendicitis
Left iliac fossa pain associated with diarrhoea with blood and mucus	Diverticulitis
Sudden onset of flank pain radiating to the groin with microscopic haematuria	Renal colic
Stools with mucus associated with abdominal pain for weeks to months	Inflammatory bowel disease

Physiology comment

Understanding how vomiting may influence both acid–base and electrolyte balance needs an understanding of the composition of the main GI secretions. Approximate values are shown in Table 3.2 opposite.

At low (unstimulated) flow rates, gastric juice contains a solution of NaCl with small amounts of H^+ and K^+. As secretion is stimulated and the flow rates increase, the secretion becomes primarily HCl with lesser amounts of K^+ and Na^+. The H^+ is actively pumped across the apical membrane into the stomach in exchange for luminal K^+ by a H^+, K^+ ATPase. Importantly, Cl^- entering the secreting parietal cell across the basolateral membrane is exchanged for HCO_3^-. The pH of the venous blood leaving the actively secreting stomach will therefore be alkaline due to the HCO_3^- added from the parietal cells.

Table 3.2 Composition of GI secretions

	Volume/ day (L)	Sodium (mmol/L)	Potassium (mmol/L)	Chloride (mmol/L)	Bicarbonate (mmol/L)	pH
Gastric secretions	1–2.5	80–20	10–20	120–150	–	2–<1
Bile (from gall bladder)	0.5	150	10	50	30	7–8
Pancreatic secretions	1.5	160	10	50–100	30–110	7–8
Small intestinal secretions	1.0	140	5	110	25	7–8

Pancreatic secretion is primarily a solution of Na^+ and Cl^- at low flow rates, but Na^+ and HCO_3^- predominate as flow rates increase. The high bicarbonate concentration of the 1–1.5 L of fluid secreted by the pancreas per day is sufficient to neutralise most of the acid entering the small intestine from the stomach. Intestinal secretions have high concentrations of Cl^- because the crypt cells that are predominantly responsible for secretion possess $Na^+K^+Cl_2$ transporters on their basolateral membranes, leading to active Cl^- secretion.

Knowing the composition of the different secretions helps explain how loss of fluid caused by vomiting from different regions of the GI tract has a range of biochemical consequences. Extensive loss of gastric secretions, through vomiting, will result in an increase in the HCO_3^- concentration of the blood and a loss of plasma chloride ions (possibly leading to hypochloraemia). This increase in HCO_3^- is caused not by the loss of H^+ from the stomach per se, but because the HCO_3^- added to the gastric circulation (the so-called alkaline tide) by the parietal cells is not neutralised as is usually the case. As the acidic chime enters the small intestine it is usually fully neutralised by HCO_3^- secretions from the pancreas and intestinal cells. The generation of HCO_3^- to supply the secretion leads to the formation of hydrogen ions and their movement into the bloodstream. If vomiting means the acidic chime does not enter the small intestine, secretion of HCO_3^- is not induced and the alkaline tide is not neutralised.

Vomiting may also produce hypovolaemia due to the loss of water and Na^+, and this fluid loss may impair the kidneys' ability to correct any acid–base disturbance present. K^+ will be lost directly in the vomit, but may also be lost in the urine as a result of the volume contraction. The volume contraction can lead to increased aldosterone levels, which act on the distal regions of the nephron to increase sodium reabsorption and also promote potassium secretion and therefore loss.

Pancreatic, intestinal and biliary secretions may be lost if vomiting occurs from below the pylorus. In this case the acid–base disturbance will be less marked than that caused by loss of primarily gastric secretions. The loss of H^+ from the stomach is balanced by HCO_3^- loss from the small intestinal fluid. Therefore these patients may well present with normal blood pH or at worst a mild metabolic alkalosis. Cl^- concentrations will also be less influenced, as the action of HCO_3^- secretion returns Cl^- as well as H^+ to the blood, balancing out the losses of these ions in the gastric secretions.

14:30 hours

After this initial assessment, the intern feels that there's enough information to present the story to the consultant.

Clinical question 3

(a) What are the key features of Jack's presentation given the information obtained so far? Before reading ahead, practise presenting his story as if you are the intern presenting to a senior colleague.

(b) What investigations (if any) do you feel are warranted? Justify your answers.

'I've just seen Jack, an 84-year-old male who lives independently and has a history of angina and has had his gall bladder and appendix out. He's had colicky abdominal pain with distension and vomiting with no bowel movements or flatus for 2 days. He's quite dehydrated and is tachycardic … I think he has a bowel obstruction and is becoming compromised … I'd like to send bloods and organise erect and supine abdominal X-rays to confirm the diagnosis and then refer him to the surgical team for admission. I'm rehydrating him and relieving his pain in the meantime.'

The consultant nods:

'Sounds sensible, excellent presentation. Maybe inserting a nasogastric tube and putting it on free drainage might make him feel more comfortable. Be sure to avoid metoclopramide as it can increase bowel motility, which is precisely what we don't want to do if he's obstructed. I'll come and review him with you once the results are back.'

He looks at the pathology request form where the intern has requested the following tests:

'FBC, ELFT, COAGS, CRP, LIPASE, AMYLASE, Ca, Mg, PO_4.'
'Hmm ? can you justify all of these tests? How would the results affect your management?'

Clinical comment

The key features of Jack's presentation are the likely diagnosis of a bowel obstruction, his clinical response to it, and identification of the underlying cause of the obstruction. The features supporting this provisional diagnosis include:

- History of vomiting and bloating, with no flatus or stools
- History of previous abdominal surgery
- Distended abdomen with reduced bowel sounds.

It is important to recognise that Jack has become compromised as a result. He is clinically dehydrated and in the early stages of hypovolaemic shock: he is tachycardic and hypotensive, with a tachypnoea suggesting attempted compensation for an underlying metabolic acidosis that results from anaerobic metabolism secondary to reduced tissue perfusion. Regardless of the ultimate diagnosis, this is a clinical condition that must be recognised early and appropriate therapy must be initiated early.

Finally, diagnosing the ultimate cause of the bowel obstruction is of paramount importance, as malignancies are a common cause of obstruction in this age group. However, this can wait until his condition has stabilised and more specific investigations such as a CT scan and a colonoscopy can be performed.

As with any condition, investigations are performed to test a specific hypothesis rather than as part of a broad fishing approach. Such an indiscriminate use of pathology and radiology testing is not only expensive, but it can create confusion and delay diagnosis if too much irrelevant information is obtained. Hence, a philosophy of asking 'How will this test affect my management? is a useful approach before requesting any investigation in any situation. In this instance:

- FBC: measures haemoglobin (an anaemia may suggest pre-existing chronic disease) and white cell count (which is a useful marker of the acute inflammatory response)
- Urea and electrolytes: after 48 hours of vomiting and fluid shifts, significant electrolyte abnormalities would be expected
- Ca, Mg, PO$_4$: these electrolytes could be abnormal in this situation
- C-reactive protein: difficult to assess how this would impact upon the diagnosis and management process, as clinical features suggest that an inflammatory process is underway
- Lipase, amylase: nothing in the history or examination suggests pancreatitis as a diagnosis, so these investigations are not indicated
- Coagulation profile: coagulation can be disturbed when a patient is acutely unwell, and if an operation is required this test is a key part of the pre-operative work-up
- Abdominal X-rays: suspected bowel obstruction is one of the few indications for plain abdominal X-rays in the era of ready access to ultrasound and CT scanning. The presence of air–fluid levels and dilated loops of bowels supports the diagnosis.

The intern crosses out the request for amylase, lipase and CRP, and sends the bloods to pathology.

15:45 hours

Jack is feeling a lot better. The 12.5 mg of morphine has relieved his pain considerably, the nasogastric tube has drained 700 mL of bile-stained fluid, and he has received 1.5 L of intravenous fluid since he arrived. His pulse rate has reduced to 96, and his blood pressure has improved to 120/75. He has had his X-rays and the blood results are back; see Figures 3.1 and 3.2, and Table 3.3 overleaf.

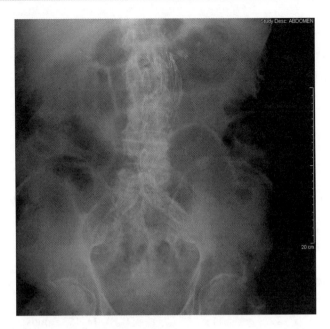

Figure 3.1 Abdominal X-ray (supine)

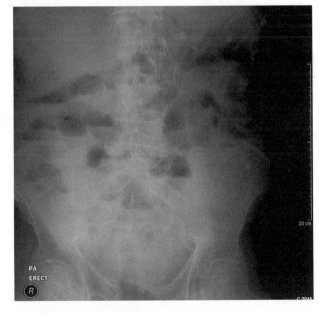

Figure 3.2 Abdominal X-ray (erect)

Table 3.3 Jack's blood results

Result	Level	Normal range
Electrolytes		
Na	149	135–145 mmol/L
K	2.7	3.5–4.5 mmol/L
Cl	91	95–110 mmol/L
HCO$_3$	32	22–32 mmol/L
Urea	3.2	3.0–8.0 mmol/L
Creatinine	0.143	< 0.120 mmol/L
Haematology		
Hb	172	115–160 g/L
WCC	13.8	4.0–11.0 × 10^9/L
Platelets	231	150–400 × 10^9/L
Coagulation profile		
PT	11 s	11–15 seconds
APTT	32 s	25–35 seconds
INR	1.0	

Physiology comment

The notable features of electrolytes in this patient are the elevated Na^+ and HCO_3^- concentrations and the lowered K^+ and Cl^- levels. The hypernatraemia can be explained by a relative excess of solute relative to extracellular water due to fluid loss through vomiting. The majority of GI secretions have a Na^+ concentration lower than that of plasma, so losses of these would result in a proportionally greater loss of water than Na^+. The reduced K^+ levels may be due to either renal losses or movement from the plasma to ICF. The elevated HCO_3^- levels indicate that the majority of the losses are from gastric secretions. These secretions are rich in H^+ and Cl^-, leading to a net excess of HCO_3^- and net reduction in total body Cl^- overall.

Clinical question 4

Describe and interpret the results. Discuss the diagnosis and the further management options. Consider how you would tell Jack the diagnosis.

The intern reviews Jack with the consultant.

'Jack, the X-rays confirm that you've got a bowel obstruction. There's a blockage that's stopping you from opening your bowels, and it's why you're bloated and vomiting so much. This could be caused by a twist in the bowel due to your previous operations, but it could also be due to a possible tumour on your bowel. There's no sign of that, and I'm not saying you've got cancer, but at your age and with an obstruction it's something that needs to be considered and looked for. Also, you've become very dehydrated and your electrolytes are quite abnormal. These will need to be corrected with intravenous fluids and close observation.'

The intern answers Jack's questions to the best of her ability and proceeds to write up further intravenous fluids and pain relief. He is referred to the surgical unit for admission.

Clinical comment

The erect and supine abdominal X-rays show the typical features of a bowel obstruction: dilated loops of bowel, and air–fluid levels. His bloods are disordered and suggest dehydration: hypernatraemia, haemocon-centration, and hypokalaemia. There is a degree of renal dysfunction and his bicarbonate is low, suggesting significant hypoperfusion. Most of these abnormalities should be corrected in a matter of days with care-ful intravenous fluid management and monitoring. Adjusting the fluid management regime in response to urine output, vital signs and clinical features of hydration is essential—under-resuscitation can be as damaging as over-resuscitation. Daily electrolyte measurement is essential in any patient receiving intravenous fluids.

Epilogue

Jack received intravenous fluids and nasogastric suction for 48 hours before signs of his obstruction began to subside. He did not require surgery to relieve the obstruction. He was restarted on clear fluids and then a normal diet, and was discharged once his bowels started working again. His daily fluid balance and his electrolytes were closely monitored, and his sodium and renal function returned to normal after 72 hours. After discharge, he was booked for an outpatient colonoscopy to look for any evidence of a bowel malignancy. Apart from finding two benign colonic polyps, this was a normal investigation.

Tips

- A suspected bowel obstruction is one of the few conditions where plain abdominal X-rays are clinically indicated.
- Request only those investigations that have the potential to alter management.
- Careful potassium replacement is necessary to replace 'third space' losses—but administer it slowly and in accordance with hospital protocols.
- Appreciate that different and competing processes often occur simultaneously to influence end electrolyte values.

References and further reading

1 Ben-Tovim, D.I., Bassham, J.E., Bennett, D.M., Dougherty, M.L. et al. Redesigning care at the Flinders Medical Centre: Clinical process redesign using 'lean thinking'. *MJA* 17 March 2008; 188 (6 Suppl): S27–31.
2 Flasar, M.H. & Goldberg, E. Acute abdominal pain. *Med Clin N Am* 2006; 90: 481–503.
3 Kamin, R.A., Nowicki, T.A., Courtney, D.S. & Powers, R.D. Pearls and pitfalls in the emergency department evaluation of abdominal pain. *Emerg Med Clin N Am* 2003; 21: 61–72.
4 Laurell, H., Hansson, L. & Gunnarsson, U. Acute abdominal pain among elderly patients. *Gerontology* 2006; 52: 339–44, doi: 10.1159/000094982
5 Martinez, J.P. & Mattu, A. Abdominal pain in the elderly. *Emerg Med Clin N Am* 2006; 24: 371–88.
6 Richardson, D.B. The access-block effect: Relationship between delay to reaching an inpatient bed and inpatient length of stay. *MJA* 2002; 177: 492–5.

Case review

Basic science questions

1 The alkaline tide is caused as a secondary consequence of:
   A HCl secretion by parietal cells
   B Pancreatic secretion
   C Biliary secretion
   D Vomiting
   E Increased plasma insulin levels

2 The pH of high flow rate gastric secretions is approximately:

  A 8

  B 7

  C 6

  D 4

  E 1

3 Vomiting from below the pylorus will generally cause:

  A Little volume loss

  B Severe metabolic alkalosis

  C Mild metabolic alkalosis

  D Marked volume loss

  E Severe respiratory alkalosis

Clinical questions

1 Match the following suspected condition with the most appropriate diagnostic investigation.

  A Bowel obstruction

  B Pancreatitis

  C Renal colic

  D Biliary colic

  E Appendicitis

  (i) Ultrasound

  (ii) Abdominal X-ray

  (iii) No investigation—clinical diagnosis

  (iv) CT abdomen

  (v) Blood tests—lipase

2 Which medication is contra-indicated in a patient with a suspected bowel obstruction?

  A Morphine

  B Fentanyl

  C Ondansetron

  D Metoclopramide

  E Potassium replacement

3 Match the following clinical features with a diagnosis of under-resuscitation (i.e. 'dry', and not enough fluids) or over-resuscitation ('wet', and fluid overload).

  A Urine output less than 30 mL / hour, tachycardic

  B Breathless, bibasal coarse crackles in the lungs

  C Widespread interstitial oedema

  D Dry mucus membranes, hypotensive

Case 4
Grace isn't herself; she looks sick …

Grace was usually a well 2-year-old girl who wouldn't be stopped by anything. But the past 3 days have exhausted her—she's off her food, she's vomiting, and she definitely does not want to go to playgroup. It's off to the emergency department tonight, as she looks sicker and her parents are very worried about her …

Clinical learning objectives

- Understand the approach to assessing an unwell child.
- Describe the common causes of acute vomiting illnesses in children.
- Describe the issues to consider when starting fluid therapy in children.
- Demonstrate how to write fluid orders and medication orders for children, based on weight.
- Know the resuscitation guidelines for children and their rationale.

Physiology learning objectives

- Outline the various triggers of the vomiting reflex.
- Describe how vomiting influences both the volume and composition of body fluid in this case.
- Discuss how coexistent volume depletion limits renal compensation of a metabolic alkalosis.

Timeline

20:15	Grace and her parents arrive at the ED; triaged as category 3 'vomiting and dehydrated'; nurse-initiated oral rehydration trial starts.
20:35	Grace vomits again in the waiting room.
21:08	Vomits again, looks more lethargic; triage category is upgraded and she is moved into a paediatric cubicle; assessment starts within the department.
21:15	Medical assessment starts; intravenous cannulation and bloods collected; fluids commenced; paediatric team notified.
22:30	Results available; Grace is feeling better; further management begins.
23:30	Grace asleep; moved to ward bed.

Clinical presentation

Grace was a well 2-year-old girl. She would usually run everywhere and had never really been sick. She didn't attend childcare but was busy almost every day attending a combination of playgroups and library activities and just simply playing with her older brother.

The past 3 days had been difficult for her and for her parents. She's been vomiting 5–6 times a day and managing to drink some fluids, but tonight she's vomited 5 times and is refusing to take anything at all. Concerned that she's becoming dehydrated, her parents wrap her in her favourite blanket and take her to the local hospital's emergency department.

20:15 hours

The family arrives at the emergency department to find a full waiting room. It is mid-winter, and the town is in the middle of an influenza outbreak. Grace has improved a little and is now looking around at this new, unfamiliar environment. She is seen by the triage nurse, who assesses her as looking a little dehydrated but not too bad. She is assigned a triage category 3 with a description of 'vomiting and dehydrated'. In keeping with the department's policy of starting treatment as early as possible and improving the patient's journey through the department, the 'dehydrated child' clinical pathway is commenced: she is given a 2 mg ondansetron wafer (an anti-emetic) and started on sips of electrolyte replacement drink. Her parents are instructed to keep note of how much fluid she drinks. Nestled in her mother's arms, she starts slowly sipping the drink provided.

Physiology comment

The vomiting response results in the evacuation of mainly the gastric contents. It involves the coordinated interaction of neural, humoral and muscular components. The reflex itself can be initiated by central or peripheral triggers that influence the central brain regions (brain stem vomiting centre and nucleus tractus solitarius) that coordinate the response. Triggers include chemicals such as opiates or pregnancy hormones that activate the chemoreceptor trigger zone, which then feeds into the central brain regions mentioned above. At a central level, the reflex can also be initiated by smells, visual stimuli, taste and somatic pain. Peripheral afferents are also able to trigger a response, especially those originating from gastric regions. Direct pharyngeal stimulation and vestibular inputs are also potent triggers for vomiting. In summary, therefore, vomiting can be a symptom of a vast number of pathologies, and it is often difficult to identify its exact cause. Once initiated, however, the act of vomiting will influence body fluid volume and composition in a predictable way.

20:35 hours

It was all going well—Grace had sipped nearly 100 mL of fluid—but then it all came back up again in one large vomit.

21:08 hours

Having just recovered from the previous vomit, she vomited again. This time, instead of crying and attempting to recover, she just lay quietly in her mother's arms. The triage sister, recognising deterioration in her condition, immediately brings her through to the treatment area as a bed in the paediatric section of the department was being prepared for her. Grace's mother lies on a bed with Grace on her lap.

Physiology comment

Vomiting is associated with the loss of water and sodium, resulting in hypovolaemia. Potassium will also be lost, because the reduced volume indirectly increases potassium loss through the distal part of the kidney nephron. The severity and pattern of the acid–base disturbance that arises as a consequence of vomiting differs, depending upon whether the vomitus arises primarily from the stomach contents or originates from below the pylorus. Prepyloric vomiting typically leads to a metabolic alkalosis and hypochloraemia. Postpyloric vomiting, on the other hand, results in only a mild metabolic alkalosis, with little change to plasma bicarbonate and chloride levels. (For further detail see Case 3.)

Clinical question 1

(a) What are the features you look for when assessing a child?
(b) Describe your approach to an unwell child who presents to your department.

Grace's assessment begins with the paediatric emergency nurse taking observations. Grace is noted to be lying quietly in her mother's arms, not interested in what's going on around her, and she doesn't seem to mind the oxygen saturation monitor being placed around her right big toe. Her observations are recorded:

- PR   170 bpm
- RR   36
- Temp   38.9°C
- 'pale, dry lips, lethargic'
- SpO_2 96%

Recognising an unwell child, the nurse applies a paediatric oxygen mask with a flow rate of 4 L per minute. Local anaesthetic cream is applied to the dorsum of both her hands and antecubital fossae in anticipation of her requiring intravenous cannulation, and the nurse proceeds to notify one of the doctors that there is a sick child in the paediatric area.

Clinical question 2

(a) What is your assessment based upon this limited information?
(b) What are the possibilities?
(c) How will you react?

Clinical comment

Assessing a child is a complex and important task—early identification of seriously ill children leads to early diagnosis and resuscitation. The absence of an obvious diagnosis must not delay the implementation of potentially life-saving therapy. As with any unwell patient, attention must be paid to the patient's ability to maintain an adequate airway, breathing and circulation. A lethargic uninterested child who is quiet is a cause for concern, and she needs urgent assessment. Simply looking at the child and assessing colour, alertness and general appearance is a good start to deciding if the child is acutely unwell and in need of urgent action. A child with a strong cry, who is well perfused and looking around, is less likely to require as urgent an intervention. Recognising abnormal vital signs is essential, and it is important to understand what the appropriate values are for the age and weight of a child. Common values for a 2-year-old girl are given in Table 4.1 below. Once the general assessment and vital signs are noted, the doctor should then expose the child fully and conduct a thorough physical examination, both looking for a cause and assessing the clinical effects of the illness.

The initial assessment of Grace would be that she is unwell and appears to be in need of resuscitation—she is quiet, pale and floppy. She appears to be clinically dehydrated, and calculating just how dehydrated can assist with setting resuscitation goals. Table 4.2 opposite details degrees of dehydration.

Sepsis from an as-yet unidentified source must be considered to be the most likely diagnosis in this instance, but other possibilities can exist concurrently, either as a cause or as a result of the underlying condition. These possibilities must be actively sought: this could be the first presentation of type 1 diabetes in the form of diabetic ketoacidosis; there could be a serious intra-abdominal cause of the symptoms; or there could be a serious metabolic abnormality present.

Table 4.1 Vitals signs for a 2-year-old

Systolic BP	75 mmHg
Heart rate	100–160 beats per minute
Respiratory rate	20–30 breaths per minute
Weight	13 kg

Table 4.2 Degrees of dehydration and clinical features

Classification	Percentage	Clinical features
Mild dehydration	< 4%	No clinical signs
Moderate dehydration	4–6%	Dry mucous membranes and sunken eyes
Severe dehydration	7–9%	Shock. Features are more pronounced with cool peripheries, decreased skin turgor, acidotic breathing

21:15 hours

The consultant is busy leading a multi-trauma resuscitation; and, therefore, asks the resident to assess the child. Noting the pale and floppy child and the vital signs already recorded, she proceeds to take a focused history:

Doctor: Is Grace usually well? Any allergies, medications, or past history?
Parent: She's a fit and well 2-year-old, no medications, and nothing to speak of ...
Doctor: Immunisations up to date?
Parent: She's had all of them.
Doctor: She's been vomiting the past few days—any diarrhoea?
Parent: No, just the vomiting. She's been completely off her food, just trying to sip water ... but then she vomits it back up soon after.
Doctor: Any fevers, rashes, sore throat, coughs, or colds?
Parent: No.
Doctor: Anyone else unwell in the house?
Parent: No—her older brother has been fine, and so have we.

The doctor proceeds to undress Grace to examine her more completely and to assess her amount of dehydration more accurately. She has dry lips and tongue, and her eyes appear sunken. Her skin is dry, and her lower limbs are cool with a capillary refill of 3 seconds. There is no rash, and chest auscultation reveals no crackles or wheezes. Her tympanic membranes and throat appear normal. Recognising a sick child in need of resuscitating, the resident and the nurse prepare to cannulate the child.

Clinical question 3

(a) What size cannula would you use?
(b) What blood tests would you request?
(c) Would you give anything through the cannula?
(d) Write down your problem list as it stands right now.

Clinical comment

Intravenous cannulation is a potentially distressing procedure for children; so the use of a local anaesthetic agent at the site of the cannulation is recommended, such as EMLA ('Eutectic Mixture of Local Anaesthetic', a mixture of lignocaine and prilocaine) or a similar product. Given Grace's lethargic state, it is unlikely she would be bothered by the procedure anyway, and time should not be spent waiting for the local anaesthetic to work if urgent intravenous access is required. An alternative is to use inhaled nitrous oxide during the procedure. A 22G cannula is a good size for a 2-year-old.

Blood tests are used to test hypotheses: to diagnose the underlying condition, and to assess the clinical effects of the condition. In this instance, with sepsis and no obvious source found, combined with what could be classed as severe dehydration, the flowing tests could be justified:

- FBC: to assess for the white cell count, a marker of inflammation
- Urea and electrolytes: to assess for any metabolic abnormality and as a baseline before starting intravenous fluids
- Glucose: children can rapidly become hypoglycaemic when acutely unwell, because they have poor glucose storage
- C-reactive protein: an inflammatory marker that can be used as a diagnostic tool
- Blood cultures: to make a definitive diagnosis if a source is not found immediately
- Venous blood gas: to provide an immediate assessment of the child's acid–base status.

Given that Grace appears to be significantly dehydrated, bordering on hypovolaemic shock, aggressive fluid resuscitation is indicated. A safe recommended starting point is a bolus of 10 mL/kg of body weight of normal saline, to be repeated based upon the clinical response. As she appears to be septic, early administration of a broad-spectrum antibiotic such as 100mg/kg of ceftriaxone is warranted.

Problem list

- Sepsis, source unknown—possible meningitis or urinary source
- Severe dehydration with shock.

Before starting any treatment, Grace is weighed while she is undressed. A chair with scales is brought to the bedside and her weight is noted to be 12.3 kg. Her mother is surprised: 'She was at least 13.5 kg just 1 week ago ...'

Grace is then cannulated with a 22G intravenous cannula in the dorsum of her left hand. Five mL of blood is drawn from the cannula, which is then secured with tape. An intravenous line of 130 mL of normal saline is set up and delivered as a bolus. The blood is placed into paediatric blood tubes and sent to the laboratory for urgent analysis. A bedside glucose test is performed, revealing the blood glucose level to be 6.2 mmol/L.

The resident presents Grace's story to the consultant.

'Grace is a previously well 2-year-old girl who's been unwell for the past 3 days, but she's worse tonight. She's been vomiting up to 6 times a day, and is off her food. She's had fevers, but no coughs, colds or rashes. She has no diarrhoea, and everyone else in the house is well. Right now she's lethargic and pale, with a temperature of 38.9°C, and she's what I think to be at least 7% dehydrated. I've cannulated her, sent bloods, and I'm just about to give her 1 g of ceftriaxone. I'm not sure what the source is, but I'm worried it could be either meningococcal disease or from her urine.'

The consultant nods in agreement:

'If you think she could have meningococcal disease, then you'd better add penicillin to the ceftriaxone ... Have you contacted the paediatric team yet?'

The resident nods. 'I'll ring the registrar now.'

Meanwhile, Grace is still looking unwell—she is still pale and cool. The consultant reviews her and suggests another 10 mL/kg bolus of fluid, just as the venous blood gas result becomes available.

Clinical question 4

(a) What results would you be expecting on the venous gas result? Interpret the results once you have considered the possibilities.

(b) What do you calculate her fluid deficit to be?

(c) How can you confirm or rule out the possible sources of infection? Why is this important?

Table 4.3 Venous blood gas result

Result	Level	Normal range
pH	7.57	7.35–7.45
pCO_2	17	35–45 mmHg
pO_2	41	N/A
HCO_3	36	24 mmol/L
Na	123	135–145 mmol/L
K	2.5	3.5–4.5 mmol/L
Lactate	4.8	< 0.8 mmol/L
Hb	18.2	105–140 g/L

Physiology note

Grace's prolonged vomiting, which is from above the pylorus, has led to a significant loss of volume and hydrogen ion, and therefore a metabolic alkalosis has developed. The lactate levels are elevated as a consequence of the reduced volume and underperfusion of the tissues, and therefore a metabolic acidosis may be expected. The prolonged vomiting and loss of acidic gastric contents is more significant, however, and so the metabolic alkalosis pattern predominates. An alkalosis develops as the HCO_3 generated by the parietal cells during acid secretion is not neutralised by the subsequent movement of the acidic gastric contents into the small intestine, and this leads to an elevated plasma HCO_3 concentration (see Case 3). Grace's tachycardia and low blood pressure indicate a significantly reduced plasma volume bordering on circulatory shock. The hypokalaemia is a direct result of the volume deficit. A small loss of potassium occurs through vomiting, but the volume deficit causes a significant increase in renal excretion of K. This occurs because the volume deficit triggers the renin–angiotensin system, leading to elevated plasma aldosterone levels. This hyperaldosterone state increases K excretion through the distal nephron.

Metabolic alkalosis with a co-existing volume depletion, as in Grace's presentation, is seen commonly. The pattern of disturbance to body fluid volume and acid–base balance may be caused by prolonged vomiting, gastric suction, and treatment with diuretics (except carbonic anhydrase and potassium-sparing types). Once there is a volume deficit and alkalosis is established, the renal system, rather than compensating and correcting the alkalosis, will act to perpetuate the imbalance by producing a 'paradoxical aciduria', the mechanism of which is discussed below.

Initially, as bicarbonate levels begin to rise, intracellular and extracellular buffers limit the effect on pH. The increased pH soon stimulates a reduction in the rate and depth of ventilation to retain more CO_2, returning the $[HCO_3] : [0.03pCO_2]$ closer to the normal 20 : 1 ratio, and therefore the accumulation of HCO_3 is compensated to some degree. The capacity for the respiratory system to compensate for the raised HCO_3 levels in this way is limited, however, because complete compensation would lead to the development of an unacceptable level of hypoxia. During respiratory compensation the breathing rate rarely slows past the point where the pCO_2 would increase above 55 mmHg.

The renal system should increase the renal excretion of filtered bicarbonate, and therefore be able to correct the underlying acid–base imbalance over a matter of hours to days. The coexistent volume depletion, however, limits the renal system's ability to excrete an alkaline urine, and an acid urine is formed inappropriately. The loss of volume and sodium triggers the renin–angiotensin system, which secondarily triggers acid secretion in the distal tubule of the nephron. Sodium is also reabsorbed avidly in the proximal tubule in response to the low body levels, with the consequent reabsorption of the filtered bicarbonate. Both these factors limit the renal system's ability to compensate for the alkalosis. In addition, the hypokalaemia that is also present will stimulate acid secretion from the distal tubular segments, contributing to perpetuation of the alkalosis. The result is the formation of an acid urine, and the kidney is unable to correct the underlying acid–base disturbance. The key approach to managing a metabolic alkalosis that has arisen due to prolonged vomiting is therefore to concentrate on re-expanding the plasma volume as quickly as possible. Once the volume deficit has been addressed, the renal system will quickly be able to excrete the bicarbonate load and correct the acid–base imbalance.

Clinical comment

Grace is dehydrated and shocked, so a metabolic acidosis might be expected. However, she has an alkalosis present, reflecting a metabolic abnormality associated with prolonged vomiting. Nevertheless she has the clinical features of poor perfusion and hypovolaemia, so these need to be addressed. As with all sick patients, a structured approach to resuscitation can help focus treating staff in their efforts—she is supporting her airway; her breathing, although rapid, is assisted with the administration of oxygen via mask; and her circulation is compromised but is being addressed by the infusion of intravenous fluids in 10 mL kg boluses.

Calculating her fluid deficit is very important and can guide appropriate fluid therapy. There are two approaches in this patient: the estimated 7% dehydration, and her possible weight loss of more than 1 kg. Based on a weight of 13.5 kg, 7% of dehydration would equate to a deficit of 945 mL. Her weight loss, which would be mostly fluid, equates to approximately 1200 mL. Replacement that is too rapid can exacerbate and create other problems, such as greater electrolyte abnormalities and dangerous fluid shifts between the interstitial and intravascular spaces; on the other hand, inadequate fluid replacement can prolong hypovolaemic shock and the consequences of poor perfusion. Fluid management will be based on replacing the deficit over an extended period—one regime suggests replacing the deficit over 24 hours, with half replaced in the first 8 hours and the rest over the remaining 16 hours. This is in addition to the ongoing fluid maintenance requirements. A sensible approach to fluid management in this child is to restore circulating volume titrated against the clinical features of capillary refill, pulse rate and conscious state, and to monitor electrolytes closely.

The source of the presumed sepsis is important, both in the short term and in the long term. A diagnosis of meningococcal disease has serious consequences for the patient as far as management and prognosis is concerned, but also has significant public health implications that may require notification to public health authorities, contact tracing and antibiotic prophylaxis. A diagnosis of a urinary tract infection, especially in a girl, has long-term consequences for the patient in that up to 35% of females with a proven urinary tract infection are found to have vesico-ureteric reflux. Missing this diagnosis can lead to scarring of the kidneys and chronic renal disease later in life.

The consultant proceeds to calculate the fluid orders:

> 'Her weight equals 13 kg, therefore her maintenance would be 4 mL/kg/hour
> for the first 10 kg, then 2 mL/kg/hour for the next 10 kg ... that would make
> it 44 mL per hour.
>
> 'Her deficit is approximately 1 L, to be replaced over 24 hours ... she's had
> 2 boluses of 130 mL already, so that leaves 740 mL to be given over the
> next 24 hours, with 370 mL over the first 8 hours (which is 46 mL/h) and
> the remaining 370 mL over 16 hours (which is 23 mL/h).'

Bearing in mind her electrolyte abnormalities and the need for volume
replacement, the consultant chooses 5% dextrose in 0.45% sodium chloride
with potassium as the maintenance fluid, and 0.9% sodium chloride ('normal
saline') as the replacement. Therefore, her fluid orders are written as shown
in Table 4.4 below.

Table 4.4 Fluid order

Date & time	Purpose	Fluid	Additives	Rate	Signed	Time started
3/12 21:45	Maintenance	1000 mL 5% dex + ½ N/S	20 mmol KCl	44 mL/ hour	Geoff Couser	21:45
3/12 21:45	Replacement	500 mL N/S		46 mL/ hour for 8 hours; then	Geoff Couser	21:45
4/12 05:45	Replacement	500 mL N/S		23 mL/ hour for 16 hours	Geoff Couser	

22:30 hours

After the two boluses totalling 260 mL of normal saline, Grace is looking a
little brighter and her colour has improved. She is starting to look around
the room and her vital signs are recorded as follows:

- PR   140 bpm
- RR   30

The pathology results become available (see Table 4.5 overleaf).

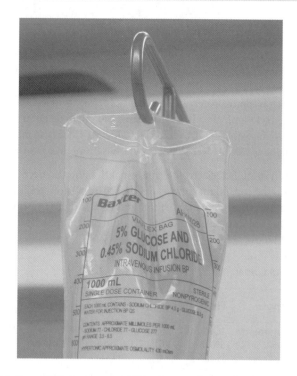

Figure 4.1 Bag of 5% dextrose / 0.45% saline ready for infusion

Table 4.5 Pathology results

Result	Level	Normal range
Na	126	135–145 mmol/L
K	2.7	3.5–4.5 mmol/L
Cl	87	95–110 mmol/L
Urea	4.5	3.0–8.0 mmol/L
Cr	0.076	< 0.120 mmol/L
CRP	234.5	< 5 mg/L
Hb	18.5	105–140 g/L
Platelets	542	150–400 × 10^9/L
WCC	18.9	4.0–11.0 × 10^9/L
Neutrophils	17.8	1.5–7.0 × 10^9/L

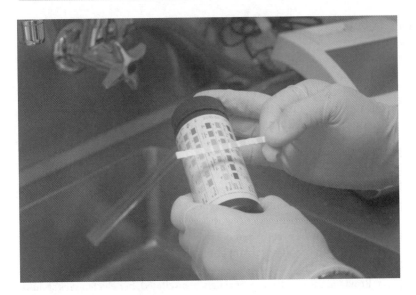

Figure 4.2 Testing the urine

An in–out urinary catheter is passed to obtain a reliable and sterile urine specimen. The urine appears cloudy and is collected in a sterile container. Before it is sent to the lab the specimen is tested in the department (see Figure 4.2 above and Table 4.6 below).

Table 4.6 Ward urine test

Leucocytes	+++
Nitrites	++
Red cells	+
Ketones	+++
Specific gravity	1.24

Clinical question 5

(a) Interpret the available results.
(b) What is the likely diagnosis?
(c) How will you manage the electrolyte abnormalities?

Clinical comment

The results are consistent with an acute inflammatory process—the white cell count is elevated, predominantly with neutrophils, and the C-reactive protein is elevated. In this instance, the CRP would not alter management, but it can play a role in tracking progress as treatment continues. The haemoglobin is elevated, suggesting dehydration. The electrolytes are consistent with the values found on the initial venous gas, which are in keeping with significant loss of Na, K, Cl and H from the GI tract.

The bedside urine test is consistent with a urinary tract infection. The sample will be sent to the pathology laboratory for microscopy and culture, which will confirm the diagnosis and guide therapy. It also makes the diagnosis of meningococcal disease less likely, as the chance of two separate diagnoses seems remote. Nevertheless, it would be prudent to continue with broad-spectrum antibiotic cover until the blood cultures yield a result.

Provided the child is appropriately resuscitated, her electrolytes should correct themselves as her body's equilibrium is restored. Given such abnormal results and the large amounts of fluid charted, the electrolytes should be repeated 6–8 hours after starting the fluids to ensure they are actually starting to correct.

23:30 hours

Grace is looking much settled. She is sleeping soundly in a bed, and her vital signs are improving: her pulse rate has settled to 130, and her respiratory rate has almost returned to normal. Her colour has improved and her peripheries are feeling much warmer than before. Her intravenous fluids have been charted and she will have another blood test at 6 a.m. to ensure that she is receiving appropriate therapy. Grace, with her mother, will be transferred to the high dependency area within the paediatric ward and will be closely monitored by nursing and medical staff overnight.

Epilogue

Grace had a comfortable night and started to take oral fluids the next day. Her 6 a.m. blood tests showed her sodium increasing to 130, her chloride over 100, and her potassium at 3.6. The rate of administration of her maintenance fluids was reduced to account for her increased oral intake and to prevent fluid overload.

Her blood cultures signalled positive for gram-negative rods early in the day, and her urine microscopy revealed an abundance of leucocytes and gram-negative rods, consistent with an *Escherichia coli* urinary infection. Grace was discharged well on oral antibiotics 48 hours later, her electrolytes having returned to normal, and with plans for outpatient investigation for possible vesico-ureteric reflux.

N Malik
hold till

2 3 JUN 2014

... that a child with isolated vomiting has 'gastro'. Vomit-
... ign of serious underlying disease that must be sought

... e actual fluid deficit serves to guide therapy, but
... hould not delay volume expansion in resuscitation.
... ren, check the electrolytes and glucose 6–8 hours after
... travenous fluid therapy, and then according to results
... cal status.
... ypotonic fluids can promote hyponatraemia through
... ssive administration of water, and therefore must be
... en replacing fluid deficits.

... and further reading

... ordan, A., Playfor, S., Millman, G. & Khader, A. Hyponatraemia ... emia during intravenous fluid administration. *Arch Dis Child* 2008; 93: 285–7.

2 Cameron, P., Jelinek, G., Everitt, I., Browne, G. & Raftos, J. (eds). *Textbook of paediatric emergency medicine*, Churchill Livingstone, Edinburgh, 2006.

3 Holliday, M.A., Ray, P.E. & Friedman, A.L. Fluid therapy for children: Facts, fashions and questions. *Arch Dis Child* 2007; 92: 546–50.

4 Hoorn, E.J., Geary, D., Robb, M., Halperin, M.L. & Bohn, D. Acute hyponatremia related to intravenous fluid administration in hospitalized children: An observational study. *Pediatrics* 2004; 113: 1279–84.

5 Ishimine, P. The evolving approach to the young child who has fever and no obvious source. *Emerg Med Clin N Am* 2007; 25: 1087–115.

6 Jacobson, S.H., Hansson, S. & Jakobsson, B. Vesico-ureteric reflux: Occurrence and long-term risks. *Acta Pædiatr* 1999; 431 Suppl: 22–30.

7 Neville, K.A., Verge, C.F., Rosenberg, A.R., O'Meara, M.W. & Walker, J.L. Isotonic is better than hypotonic saline for intravenous rehydration of children with gastroenteritis: A prospective randomised study, *Arch Dis Child* 2006; 91: 226–32.

Case review

Basic science questions

1 A metabolic alkalosis with a co-existing volume depletion caused by vomiting leads to:
   A A paradoxical acid urine
   B A paradoxical alkaline urine
   C Inactivation of the renin–angiotensin system
   D Increased total body sodium levels
   E Effective renal compensation

2 Hypokalaemia is often associated with vomiting and is caused by:
   A Increased dietary intake
   B Inactivation of the renin–angiotensin system
   C Increased renal tubular excretion
   D ECF expansion
   E Inactivation of the potassium transporters in the thick ascending limb of the Loop of Henle

3 The vomiting reflex can be triggered by which of the following?
   A Smell
   B Opiates
   C Visual stimuli
   D Vestibular input
   E All of the above

Clinical questions

1 Match the following symptoms and signs of an infective process with the most likely diagnosis in a child.
   A Fever, offensive urine, and vomiting.
   B Lethargic infant, febrile, and purpuric rash.
   C Breathlessness, cough, and wheeze in a 6-month-old.
   D Bulging right tympanic membrane with pain and fever.
      (i) Bronchiolitis
      (ii) Meningococcal sepsis
      (iii) Otitis media
      (iv) Urinary tract infection

2 Which of the following fluids should not be used in intravenous rehydration in children?
   A 0.9% saline
   B 5% dextrose
   C 5% dextrose with 0.45% saline
   D 3% dextrose with 0.33% saline

3 Match the following clinical features with the degree of dehydration in a child.

   A Cool peripheries, decreased skin turgor, and acidotic breathing.
   B Dry mucous membranes and sunken eyes.
   C Vomiting and diarrhoea, normal vital signs, and the child looks well.
   D Pulse rate 190, lethargic, capillary refill 5 seconds, and dry parched lips.

      (i) 1–3%
     (ii) 4–6%
    (iii) 7%
     (iv) 9–10%

Case 5
My husband's got terrible pain in his belly and now he's collapsed ... I need an ambulance now!

And so began the 000 call. Craig was usually in good health, but now he's in an ambulance en route to the hospital, after having complained of back pain and then collapsing ... He's recovered a little, and he'll be here in 5 minutes.

Clinical learning objectives

- Be able to recognise the clinical features of shock and how to institute appropriate emergency management regardless of the cause.
- Describe the causes of life-threatening abdominal pain and how they are diagnosed rapidly in the emergency department.
- Understand how time-critical processes can be activated quickly in life-threatening situations.
- Understand how bedside investigations in the emergency department can be used to facilitate diagnosis and management.

Physiology learning objectives

- Define shock and describe the various cardiovascular responses to hypovolaemic shock.
- Understand the physiological basis for fluid shifts from one body fluid compartment to another as a consequence of hypovolaemic shock.
- Outline the theoretical advantage of using colloid versus crystalloid therapy to re-expand the plasma volume.
- Understand the mechanisms by which the renal system minimises fluid and electrolyte loss during shock (renal success).
- Describe the process by which ischaemically mediated acute renal failure develops.
- Explain the biochemistry results seen in this case.

Timeline

16:30	Craig complains of the sudden onset of left flank pain; soon after he feels weak and collapses; his wife calls an ambulance.
16:39	Ambulance on scene, crew commences treatment.
16:46	Departs house, notifies emergency department of estimated time of arrival and current condition.
16:55	Arrives in emergency department; assessment continues.
17:13	Change in condition.
17:25	Leaves emergency department; pathology results available.
17:35	Arrives in operating theatre (OT).

Clinical presentation

Craig was a reasonably well 79-year-old male who lived comfortably and independently at home with his wife. He kept himself busy by volunteering for the local Meals on Wheels group and looking after his wife. He had a history of high blood pressure and was on 2 antihypertensives. Two years earlier he had suffered a transient ischaemic attack, for which he was on aspirin.

16:30 hours

Craig was watering the garden when he felt a severe pain in his left lower back. He'd never had such bad pain before, and he began sweating profusely. He called out to his wife, and started to move indoors, but before he could make it inside he collapsed. His wife promptly called the ambulance and anxiously awaited their arrival.

16:39–16:46 hours

Based upon the call 'My husband's collapsed and not moving', a paramedic crew is dispatched as a category 1 response. Arriving on the scene 9 minutes after the call, the paramedics find a semi-conscious elderly male lying on the garden path. He responds to initial questions but is unwilling to stand up. He indicates that he has severe pain in his left flank region. The paramedics record the vital signs as they load him on to the stretcher and prepare to transport him to hospital. They are:

- PR   110 bpm
- BP   90/60
- RR   26
- '… cool peripheries'

Wasting little time, they proceed to the nearest hospital. Intravenous cannulation with an 18G cannula is performed en route, and 2.5 mg of intravenous morphine is given for his ongoing severe left flank pain. A 500 mL bag of 0.9% saline is prepared and a slow infusion is commenced.

Clinical question 1

(a) Based upon the information provided so far, what are the possible diagnoses?
(b) What are the management priorities at this time?

16:55 hours

The ambulance arrives at the emergency department. By now Craig is feeling much better—his pain has eased significantly, and he almost feels 'back to my usual self'. He had received 5 mg of morphine and approximately 250 mL of the intravenous normal saline. He is assigned a triage category 2 as 'left flank pain and collapse, ?renal colic' and is transferred on to a bed in a cubicle. His nursing assessment commences and he is quickly seen by the consultant, who also commences an assessment. The following vital signs are recorded:

- PR   120 bpm
- BP   100/60
- RR   28
- GCS   15
- In pain

The patient looks unwell, and is noted to be sweaty with cool peripheries. A focused examination is performed. The consultant notes that the patient is tender in the peri-umbilical region, and a palpable pulsatile mass is looked for and found.

Clinical question 2

(a) What is the diagnosis?
(b) What should be done now? Describe your actions.

Clinical comment

The clinical scenario of an elderly patient with collapse and flank pain should alert medical and paramedical staff to the likely diagnosis of a leaking or ruptured abdominal aortic aneurysm. This is a true surgical emergency, and time should not be wasted waiting for radiological or pathological investigations that will delay the diagnosis and definitive management. Urgent referral to the vascular surgical team is required even on a suspicion of the condition, as early notification can facilitate emergency care by allowing for re-scheduling of theatre time and arranging an intensive care bed.

A leaking aneurysm can present with signs and symptoms similar to renal colic; hence, a leaking abdominal aortic aneurysm ('AAA') must be considered in any elderly patient presenting with back pain or flank pain. There are some important clues in this patient's presentation that there is a more sinister diagnosis present: the history of collapse, the presence of a tachycardia, a blood pressure that is low for a patient known to have hypertension, and tachypnoea. This last sign is of critical importance as it is often the first sign of shock: the pathophysiological process underlying this clinical sign is likely to be a metabolic acidosis resulting from poor perfusion, and the tachypnoea is present as the body attempts to compensate by increasing the respiratory rate and 'blowing off' carbon dioxide. Management is then geared towards making the appropriate referrals and transporting the patient to the operating theatre as quickly as possible.

Physiology comment

Shock can be defined as inadequate tissue perfusion as a result of depressed cardiac output. Shock can be usefully categorised based upon the cause of the drop in cardiac output:

- Hypovolaemic (low circulating volume)
- Cardiogenic (decreased cardiac performance)
- Distributive (normal blood volume but vasodilation)
- Obstructive (impediment to blood flow).

In this case the patient is obviously experiencing haemorrhagic shock (a subset of hypovolaemic shock). Compensation in hypovolaemic shock is often initially successful. Increased sympathetic outflow via the baroreceptor reflex leads to increased heart rate and contractility, and increased peripheral resistance leading to shunting of blood centrally. Remember that, even though the total peripheral resistance may increase, the resistance of the coronary and cerebral arteries may well decrease to ensure adequate perfusion to these crucial areas.

Concerned that the patient has a leaking AAA which has temporarily stopped bleeding, the management priorities change rapidly. Two large-bore 16 gauge intravenous cannulae are inserted and blood is simultaneously taken for a cross-match of 10 units of packed cells, full blood count, urea and electrolytes, and a coagulation profile. A venous blood gas is performed in the emergency department at the same time. The vascular surgical registrar is contacted and asked to come urgently to review the patient, and the operating theatres are notified that the patient may need to proceed there urgently.

Physiology comment

Determinants of fluid flow across capillary wall

Net fluid movement out of the capillaries is equal to the filtration coefficient (Kf) × net filtration pressure (NFP). The water permeability and surface area of the capillaries determines Kf, and NFP is determined by the balance of the Starling forces acting across the capillary wall. The following factors therefore determine the rate of fluid movement from the capillaries (plasma compartment) into the interstitial space:

1 rate of filtration:
   - capillary forces—hydrostatic and osmotic
   - capillary permeability
   - capillary surface area
2 rate of reabsorption:
   - lymphatic system.

Fluid movement from the interstitial space into the capillaries is favoured if there is a decrease in capillary pressure, increase in interstitial pressure, increase in plasma oncotic pressure or decrease in interstitial oncotic pressure. The arterial hypotension brought about by the loss of blood, and the arteriolar constriction due to the baroreceptor-mediated shock response lowers the hydrostatic pressure in the capillaries. The balance of the Starling forces therefore promotes the net reabsorption of interstitial fluid into the vascular compartment. Upwards of 1 L per hour can move from the interstitial spaces into the circulation after acute blood loss. The plasma colloid pressure will decline during this period as a consequence of the diluting effect of the interstitial fluid on the plasma constituents.

Adequate restoration of intravascular volume is vitally important in managing the shocked patient. The administered fluid may stay in the intravascular compartment or equilibrate with the interstitial/intracellular fluid compartments. The primary goal of volume administration is to establish stable haemodynamics by restorating circulating plasma volume as rapidly as possible. However, excessive fluid accumulation, particularly in the interstitial tissue, should be minimised. Traditional crystalloid hypotonic (e.g. dextrose in water), isotonic (e.g. lactated Ringer's solution) and hypertonic solutions (e.g. 7.5% saline solution) will expand both the plasma and interstitial compartments to varying degrees. This occurs as, once administered, the solute passes freely across the capillary endothelium along with water until an appropriate equilibrium is established.

Protein, however, is unable to pass easily across the capillary wall, and this ensures that any protein added to the plasma will remain in only the plasma compartment. As discussed earlier, the colloid osmotic pressure is a key determinant of the Starling equation that acts to retain fluid in the plasma compartment. Administration of colloid fluid replacement products therefore promises to re-expand the plasma volume quickly while minimising interstitial expansion, and is at least theoretically attractive.

A review of the present literature indicates that it has not been proven that colloid therapy is any more effective in terms of patient outcomes than using crystalloid solutions. The choice of fluid therapy, however, does impact upon coagulation, cost, immune and organ function. It has been argued that these potential side-effects associated with fluid administration should be the main consideration when choosing the most appropriate fluid to use (Boldt, 2005), rather than a theoretical consideration of how the therapy would influence the prevailing Starling forces.

Clinical question 3

Discuss the role of intravenous fluid resuscitation in this situation.

Clinical comment

Intravenous fluid resuscitation has been the mainstay of the management of shocked hypotensive patients for many decades, the rationale being that the fluid restores circulating blood volume and maintains vital organ perfusion while definitive management is being arranged. There may, however, be unintended consequences in selected cases: if the internal bleeding has been contained by tamponade, then a surge in blood pressure may dislodge the clot and re-start the bleeding. It is likely that this is what has happened with Craig's abdominal pain and collapse—his aorta has ruptured, causing hypovolaemic shock, and this has allowed time for a clot to form and prevent further bleeding. Is there a role for further intravenous fluids at this stage? Probably not—even though he is tachycardic, hypotensive and has cool peripheries, he is conscious. This suggests that his brain is being adequately perfused. Rather than focusing on a blood pressure measurement of 90/70 in isolation, understanding and assessing the clinical features of perfusion are of paramount importance. In this case, if Craig is to survive, his best chance is to make it to the operating theatre alive so that a vascular surgeon can operate and repair the aorta. Similar principles apply to the management of suspected ruptured ectopic pregnancies.

Should Craig deteriorate in the meantime and become unconscious, then staff must be prepared to aggressively resuscitate using accepted protocols of intravenous fluid and blood products while the patient is being transferred to the operating theatre.

As the patient is being prepared for an anticipated transfer to the operating theatre, the emergency physician performs a bedside ultrasound scan (see Figure 5.1).

Clinical question 4

(a) What is the value of the use of ultrasound in the emergency department? What are the alternatives?

(b) Interpret the venous gas. How reliable is it compared to an arterial blood gas?

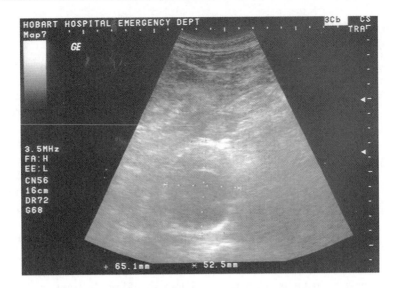

Figure 5.1 Ultrasound image of AAA

The venous blood gas result is available, with the results shown in Table 5.1 below.

Table 5.1 Venous blood gas results

Result	Level	Normal range
pH	7.23	7.36–7.44
pCO2	13 mmHg	35–45 mmHg
pO2	42 mmHg	N/A
HCO3	16 mmol/L	22–32 mmol/L
Hb	92 g/L	130–165 g/L
Lactate	5.8 mmol/L	< 0.8 mmol/L
Na	136 mmol/L	135–145 mmol/L
K	5.9 mmol/L	3.5–4.5 mmol/L

Clinical comment

Bedside ultrasound has a number of applications in the emergency department, and it has become well established in trauma management and other circumstances. It has been proven to be useful and staff can be readily trained in its use. This scan clearly shows a 6.5 × 5.2 cm aortic aneurysm, with a crescent-shaped thrombus located anteriorly.

The use of bedside ultrasound in this situation is limited only to identifying the presence or absence of an aneurysm—it is unable to determine accurately if it has ruptured or not. The clinical features of a ruptured aneurysm combined with the aneurysm confirmed on ultrasound are enough to make the diagnosis. Computerised tomography scanning of the abdomen can display the extent of the rupture and its more precise location, but the disadvantage lies in transferring an unstable patient away from the resuscitation area to a remote part of the hospital where continued resuscitation is often difficult. In general, unstable patients of whatever aetiology should not be transferred for CT scanning.

The key acid-base information provided by a venuos blood gas is not remarkably different from values derived from an arterial blood gas. The pO_2 is of course expected to be different from arterial values but pH, HCO_3 and pCO_2 values will be similar enough to the arterial gas assessment, with the pH being marginally lower and the HCO_3 and pCO_2 being slightly higher due to the dissolved CO_2 in venuos blood compared to arterial blood. The information provided can reliably inform treating clinicians about the patient's acid-base status without causing additional discomfort or spending the additional time needed to obtain an arterial sample.

17:13 hours

The patient has been reviewed by the vascular registrar, who agrees that the patient should proceed to theatre immediately. As she departs to prepare for the operation with her consultant, Craig deteriorates. He becomes less responsive, and will only open his eyes to painful stimulus. His pulse rate has increased to 140 and his blood pressure is 70/40.

Clinical question 5

What is your response?

Clinical comment

Craig has been compensating reasonably well until now, but now it appears that he can no longer do so—he is decompensating. He is showing obvious clinical features of poor perfusion, and hence aggressive resuscitation is necessary in order to deliver him to the operating theatre alive. Having two large-bore IV cannulae in place in anticipation of such deterioration is essential, as now is not the time to be trying to obtain difficult intravenous access. It is also essential to have blood products ready to use at the bedside should such a deterioration occur. Staff should always be looking ahead and anticipating problems and prepare for them before they happen.

In this circumstance, addressing the ABCs is paramount—maintain the Airway, support Breathing, and restore Circulation. Remember, the aim is to keep the patient alive until he can make it to theatre and receive definitive surgical management. The ideal fluid to use would be properly typed packed cells. If they are not available, then commence resuscitation with 0.9% saline and then use O negative blood (the 'universal donor'). Much has been written about using either crystalloid fluids (such as 0.9% normal saline, or Hartmann's solution) or colloids (such as Haemaccel, or Gelofusine), but in reality there is very little difference in their use in an acute setting such as this.

The team responds in a coordinated and structured manner. One doctor provides chin lift and applies a bag-valve-mask apparatus to Craig's face, thus providing airway and breathing support; and two bags of O negative blood are rapidly infused, one through each 16G intravenous cannula. Craig's mental state improves after about two minutes of resuscitation, indicating improved end-organ perfusion, and theatre is notified that the patient has deteriorated and is proceeding there immediately. As he departs, his blood results become available (see Table 5.2 overleaf).

Table 5.2

Result	Level	Normal range
Biochemistry		
Na	137	135–145 mmol/L
K	5.8	3.5–4.5 mmol/L
Cl	100	95–110 mmol/L
HCO_3	13	22–32 mmol/L
Urea	14.6	3.0–8.0 mmol/L
Creatinine	0.193	< 0.120 mmol/L
Haematology		
Hb	97	130–180 g/L
WCC	18.5	$4.0–11.0 \times 10^9$/L
Platelets	345	$150–400 \times 10^9$/L
Coagulation profile		
PT	13 s	11–15 seconds
APTT	32 s	25–35 seconds
INR	1.2	

Physiology comment

Acute renal success

Loss of fluid and electrolytes is reduced during haemorrhage in response to the reduced arterial pressure. Anti-diuretic hormone (ADH) is released from the posterior pituitary in large amounts due to baroreceptor-mediated sympathetic outflow. Anti-diuretic hormone acts on the late distal tubule and collecting duct, increasing the permeability of these sites to water. Water therefore passes from the tubule into the kidney interstitium, producing a low-volume concentrated urine. High levels of ADH also have a potent vasoconstrictor effect on smooth muscle, helping to augment the systemic increase in total peripheral resistance elicited by the shock response.

A combination of reduced cardiovascular pressures and reduced flow to the distal nephron stimulates the release of renin, activating the renin–angiotensin system (RAAS). Increased circulating renin increases the level of angiotensin two, which has both a potent vasoconstrictor effect itself and causes the release of aldosterone. Aldosterone acts primarily on the late distal tubule and collecting ducts, increasing sodium reabsorption in these regions. This avid active reabsorption of sodium leads to the passive reabsorption of water, reducing both salt and water loss. This reflex reduction in urine volume indicates that the kidney is responding appropriately to the lowered systemic pressure brought about by blood loss, and should not be viewed as a pathological process. In effect this minimisation of water and salt loss through the kidney can be viewed as 'acute renal success'.

Acute renal failure

If, however, the blood loss is severe and or prolonged, the kidney is susceptible to ischaemically mediated damage. This in itself is somewhat paradoxical, in that the kidneys receive close to 20% of resting cardiac output and are relatively small in size (roughly the size of a bar of soap). The kidneys display a low arterial venous oxygen difference, suggesting that above-average oxygen usage in not the reason the kidneys are damaged during prolonged shock. The explanation lies in the uneven distribution of blood throughout the kidney. The renal cortex (where filtration takes place) is well perfused, and initially is often little affected during shock. The deep medulla, however, is poorly perfused, even in health, and the cells associated with the thick ascending limb of the Loop of Henle can be viewed as being critically hypoxic even in health. The deep medullary regions are poorly perfused to protect and maintain the solute load in this region that is established by the countercurrent multiplier system of the Loop of Henle. The blood vessels associated with this region are sparse and anatomically matched with the Loops of Henle to prevent solute being carried away from the region. The solute plays a vital role as it enables water to be drawn out of the collecting ducts, enabling a concentrated urine to be formed.

In the early stages of hypovolaemic shock, the reduced arterial pressure leads to a direct reduction in driving pressure and therefore a direct reduction in blood flow. The reflex response to shock, as previously detailed (see acute renal success), is to minimise urinary losses through vasoconstriction, leading to a reduced GFR. If prolonged, acute renal success can tip over into acute renal failure as the regions of the nephron in the medulla become starved of blood and therefore of oxygen. The thick ascending limb cells are the first to fail, leading initially to a loss in renal concentrating ability and eventually to anuria.

17:25–17:35 hours

The patient is escorted to the operating theatres, where the anaesthetic and surgical teams receive handover from the emergency department team and the operation begins.

Clinical summary

This patient presented with both diagnostic and management dilemmas. The diagnosis became apparent on careful consideration of the history and performance of a focused examination, and this then allowed for rapid confirmation and rapid and appropriate management. The role of the emergency department staff is to keep the patient alive and to facilitate early definitive management. This occurred in this instance, and there were no distracters such as requests to perform a time-wasting CT scan or to wait for the blood tests to become available. These clearly would not influence the diagnosis or the management.

Ruptured aortic aneurysm is a condition associated with a high mortality, up to 100% if 3 or more variables are present on the Hardman index (based on Hb < 9, Cr > 90, age > 76, in-hospital loss of consciousness, and features of ischaemia on ECG). Based on the Hardman index, Craig was facing a high risk of mortality and his survival could not be expected. This would need to be considered if he was shocked and did not respond to resuscitation—the treating doctors would need to decide to provide palliative care in the emergency department rather than futile surgical care. Obviously such decisions are made by the most experienced doctors available, and in full and open consultation with the patient and his family.

Physiology comment

A lactic acidosis is defined as a metabolic acidosis with a pH < 7.35 and a plasma lactate greater than 7 mmol/L, as seen in this case. The tissue hypoxia caused by the haemorrhage and widespread sympathetic response lead to the metabolic production of lactate at a much greater rate than it can be recycled. The bicarbonate levels are reduced by the action of the carbonic acid–bicarbonate buffer system. The hyperkalaemia is associated with the acidosis and also with reduced renal excretion. The acidaemia also stimulates respiration, and the consequent lowering of the pCO_2 returns the pH towards normal. The elevated urea and creatinine levels are a consequence of the reduced glomerular filtration rate and therefore reduced renal excretion of these substances.

Epilogue

The patient underwent the successful emergency repair of his aneurysm and was transferred to the intensive care unit post-operatively. He remained there for 2 days before being transferred to a general surgical ward, and was discharged home 10 days later.

Tips—hypovolaemic shock

- There is more to the assessment of the shocked patient than just blood pressure—peripheral perfusion, urine output and conscious state are important signs to assess.
- The use of crystalloid fluid for resuscitation is acceptable in the initial stages, with no evidence supporting the use of colloids.
- A metabolic acidosis arises as a result of poor perfusion.
- Remember that fluid resuscitation only serves to 'buy time' while definitive management is being organised rapidly.

References and further reading

1 Bickell, W.H., Wall, M.J. Jr, Pepe, P.E., Martin, R.R. et al. Immediate versus delayed fluid resuscitation for hypotensive patients with penetrating torso injuries. *N Engl J Med* 27 Oct 1994; 331 (17): 1105–9.
2 Dent, B., Kendall, R.J., Boyle, A.A. & Atkinson, P.R.T. Emergency ultrasound of the abdominal aorta by UK emergency physicians: A prospective cohort study. *Emerg Med J* 2007; 24: 547–9.
3 Malatesha, G., Singh, N.K., Bharija, A. et al. Comparison of arterial and venous pH, bicarbonate, pCO_2 and pO_2 in initial emergency department assessment. *Emerg Med J* 2007; 24: 569–71.
4 Sakalihasan, N., Limet, R. & Defawe, O.D. Abdominal aortic aneurysm. *Lancet* 2005; 365: 1577–89.
5 Tambyraja, A.L., Murie, J.A., Chalmers, T.R.A. Prediction of outcome after abdominal aortic aneurysm rupture. *J Vasc Surg* 2008; 47: 222–30.

Case review

Basic science questions

1   Cardiogenic shock is shock caused by:
   A   Low circulating volume
   B   Decreased cardiac performance
   C   Normal blood volume but vasodilation
   D   Impediment to blood flow
   E   Loss of peripheral resistance
2   Which statement regarding ADH is most correct?
   A   ADH increases water permeability of the late distal tubule collecting ducts
   B   ADH reduces water permeability of the late distal tubule collecting ducts
   C   ADH is released from the adrenal medulla
   D   An increased ECF leads to the release of ADH
   E   ADH reduces water permeability of the proximal tubule
3   Hypovolaemic shock can lead to the development of what type of acid–base disorder?
   A   Respiratory acidosis
   B   Respiratory alkalosis
   C   Metabolic acidosis
   D   Respiratory acidosis
   E   No acid base disturbance

Clinical questions

1   Which of the following clinical features are least likely to suggest a diagnosis of a leaking aortic aneurysm?
   A   Sudden onset of abdominal pain and collapse in a 66-year-old male
   B   Left flank pain radiating around to the left groin
   C   Hypotension and a pulsatile abdominal mass
   D   Right flank pain and haematuria in a 24-year-old male
2   Match the following clinical scenarios to the suggested management options.

Clinical scenarios

   A   78-year-old female, sudden onset of abdominal pain at home, but arrives at hospital in cardiac arrest despite aggressive fluid resuscitation en route to hospital. Bedside ultrasound shows an AAA 7 cm in diameter.

B 67-year-old male, epigastric pain with a pulsatile mass, and normal vital signs.

C 78-year-old female with collapse and a pulsatile abdominal mass, arrives at hospital conscious with a blood pressure of 100/60 and a pulse rate of 110.

D 74-year-old male with collapse and a pulsatile abdominal mass, deteriorates en route and arrives at hospital semi-conscious with a blood pressure of 80/40 and a pulse rate of 140.

Management options

(i)   Notify vascular surgical team, obtain large-bore IV access, and arrange urgent CT scan of abdomen.

(ii) Notify vascular surgical team, obtain large-bore IV access, give no intravenous fluids at this stage and proceed directly to the operating theatre.

(iii) Notify vascular surgical team, obtain large-bore IV access, commence fluid resuscitation with 1 L of normal saline and O negative blood and proceed directly to the operating theatre.

(iv) Withdraw any further resuscitation efforts and explain to the family that nothing can be done.

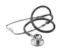

Case 6
John was hit hard by the flu ...

John had been coughing for the past few days and wasn't getting better. However, it felt like more than that, and today when he complained of pains in his belly and started vomiting, he knew it was time to seek help ...

Clinical learning objectives

- Be able to assess causes of tachypnoea in an unwell patient.
- Describe how to assess hydration status and institute immediate therapy in an acutely unwell patient.
- Justify the choice of fluid when commencing intravenous therapy.
- Discuss the causes of acute acid–base and electrolyte disturbances.

Physiology learning objectives

- Outline the role and function of glucose and insulin in metabolism.
- Describe the physiological effects of diabetic ketoacidosis (DKA) on acid–base balance and body hydration.
- Explain the physiological basis of the presenting signs of rapid breathing, increased urine output, metabolic acidosis, increased blood glucose levels (BGL), as well as the presence of glucose and ketones in the urine.
- Explain how DKA can lead to dehydration and ultimately hypovolaemic shock.
- Describe the physiological basis of the approach taken to manage DKA appropriately.

Timeline

07:40	John feels unwell after standing up and he collapses, partner calls ambulance
08:25	Ambulance arrives; records vital signs; commences limited therapy
08:50	Arrives in hospital; triaged category 3 as 'fever, dehydrated, collapse? cause'
08:55	Nursing and medical assessment commenced
09:10	Investigations ordered; diagnosis made; initial therapy started.

Clinical presentation

John had been feeling unwell for the past few days. Like many of his friends, he had recently come down with what he had self-diagnosed as a bad case of the flu, and he had been treating himself with throat lozenges, over-the-counter cold and flu tablets, and lots of water. He wasn't feeling any better after a couple of days, so he rang in sick and decided to stay in bed. Twenty-four hours of bed rest and support from his partner made little difference; in fact, he felt he was getting worse. He was increasingly thirsty and felt dehydrated despite increasing his oral intake, and his partner noticed that he was breathing faster.

07:40 hours

When he got out of bed to go to the toilet the next morning and promptly collapsed, his partner checked he was still breathing, placed him into the coma position and called an ambulance. He regained consciousness only a few seconds later but was still feeling drowsy. He lay on his side until the ambulance arrived.

08:25 hours

The ambulance arrived, and paramedics assessed the situation, recording the following observations:

- PR   120 bpm
- BP   100/50
- RR   30
- Temp   37.8°C

The paramedics placed an oxygen mask and started oxygen therapy at 10 L per minute. They obtained intravenous access in his right antecubital fossa, and, noting that he was dehydrated, started a 500 mL bag of 0.9% normal saline. John was placed onto the ambulance trolley and transported to the nearest hospital. He was alert and talking by now, and was able to recount his history to the paramedics. He added that he was usually in excellent health and on no medication.

08:50 hours

John arrives at the hospital, and is transferred immediately to a bed in a vacant cubicle. He is feeling a little better after the 500 mL of the intravenous fluid administered by the paramedics, but he is still breathless and feels very weak.

Clinical question 1

Based upon the information provided so far, what are the possible diagnoses?

Clinical comment

In this instance, a number of possibilities exist: his tachypnoea and fever could indicate developing lung sepsis. He could have an underlying dysrhythmia causing his syncopal event. Collapse and breathlessness may suggest a diagnosis of pulmonary embolism. At this stage it is too early to have a true idea as to what is wrong with John and an appropriately directed history and examination should yield more information. Most nurses and doctors, however, tend to form ideas and theories within the first few seconds of meeting a patient, and this can either ultimately prove to be correct or close minds to alternative diagnoses as more information becomes available. This phenomenon must be recognised so that appropriate treatment or management are not delayed. Emergency departments take on a huge responsibility in assessing and 'labelling' patients, and it can take time and courage to challenge a decision previously made. Caution is required before determining a diagnosis.

08:55 hours

The nurse commences his assessment and takes a set of observations that are similar to those taken by the ambulance crew. The oxygen is continued and 10 mL of blood is collected in anticipation of pathology tests being requested. The empty 500 mL bag of fluid is replaced with a 1 L bag of normal saline and commenced at a slow rate of infusion.

The intern enters the cubicle a short time later and commences the medical assessment. John is able to give a history, and the following history is recorded:

- Four days of cough and breathlessness
- Increasing lethargy and malaise
- Denies chest pain
- No headaches or neck stiffness
- Feels very thirsty, with a very dry mouth—has been trying to drink water but cannot quench thirst
- No dysuria, but has been passing a lot of urine
- No diarrhoea
- Occasional nausea with crampy central abdominal pain
- Difficulty mobilising in the past 24 hours due to feeling faint upon standing.

A physical examination is performed, but while the doctor was taking the history he noticed that John was breathing very fast and very deeply, with

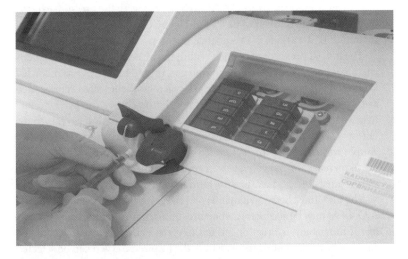

Figure 6.1 Injecting a sample into the blood gas machine for analysis

a respiratory rate of 30 breaths per minute and with an oxygen saturation of 95% on 10 litres of oxygen per minute. Keen to obtain the true status of John's respiratory function, the doctor performs an arterial blood gas (see Figure 6.1) prior to any further examination.

Clinical question 2

(a) With the history provided and the limited physical findings available, what would you expect to see on the ABG result? How can the ABG assist with diagnosis?

(b) Consider what other relevant investigations you would request that could aid your diagnosis.

Clinical comment

It is important to understand that there are two components to breathing: oxygenation, and ventilation. The two are related via the alveolar gas equation:

$$p_AO_2 = FIO_2 \, (p_{atm} - \text{water vapour}) - pCO_2/R$$

where: p_AO_2 is the partial pressure of oxygen within the alveoli, FIO_2 is the fractional concentration of inspired oxygen (0.21 breathing room air); p_{atm} is atmospheric pressure (760 mmHg at sea level); the pressure exerted by water vapour is taken to be 47 mmHg; pCO_2 is the partial pressure of carbon dioxide; and R is a resistance factor, usually taken to be 0.8.

The partial pressure of oxygen within the alveoli can be readily calculated from data from an arterial blood gas, provided the FIO_2 is recorded accurately: then the alveolar–arterial oxygen gradient (often represented as $p_{(A-a)}O_2$) can be calculated. Hyperventilation causes the pCO_2 to fall; hypoventilation causes the pCO_2 to rise. The gas equation reveals that a fall in pCO_2 will increase the alveolar oxygen partial pressure. Another simple way of saying this is that if you're hypoxic, you breathe faster to try to increase the oxygen levels in your alveoli and hence in your blood. This is a feasible explanation for John having a respiratory rate of 30.

The FIO_2 must be known to interpret the arterial blood gas accurately. A p_AO_2 of 90 may be acceptable when breathing room air, but is dangerously low if the patient is breathing 100% oxygen. The FIO_2 can be calculated easily by using a Venturi mask, where the inspired oxygen can be selected easily, but must be calculated if a low flow (or 'Hudson' mask) is being used.

John is breathing at 30 breaths a minute with an estimated tidal volume of 700 mL, producing a minute volume of 21 L. John is receiving 10 L of oxygen a minute (FIO_2 of 1.0), with an additional 11 L of room air oxygen (FIO_2 of 0.21) being drawn into his lungs each minute. Therefore, his inspired oxygen at this respiratory rate can be calculated as:

$$\frac{1.0 \times 10 + 0.21 \times 11}{21} = 0.58$$

This shows how the same flow rate of oxygen produces significantly different inspired oxygen concentrations at different minute volumes. This is important when the amount of inspired oxygen is of critical importance, such as in patients with emphysema with carbon dioxide retention.

However, hyperventilation can also be caused by (and can produce, for that matter) acute acid–base disturbances. The Henderson–Hasselbach equation can explain this:

$$H_2O + CO_2 \Leftrightarrow H_2CO_3 \Leftrightarrow H^+ + HCO_3^-$$

An accumulation of carbon dioxide caused by an underlying acidosis promotes hyperventilation as the body tries to compensate and remove the carbon dioxide via the respiratory system. Therefore, hyperventilation may be the result of an underlying acidotic process rather than purely a respiratory symptom or sign alone. The arterial blood gas can reveal any such abnormality.

Given John's clinical state, he could have an elevated alveolar–arterial oxygen gradient, representing consolidation in his chest, or he could have an underlying metabolic acidosis, where the hyperventilation represents his attempts at compensation. Of course, both processes could be occurring simultaneously. This would be represented by a low pH, a low pCO_2, and a low pO_2. The presence of such features should alert staff to actively seek the possible causes of such effects.

09:10 hours

While waiting for the results of the arterial blood gas, the intern proceeds to examine John. Noting his mucous membranes are dry and the history of his excessive thirst, she assesses him to be significantly dehydrated, and immediately asks that a 1 L bag of normal saline be infused over 1 hour. Although he is tachypnoeic and febrile, there are no added sounds in his chest. His abdomen is soft, with mild tenderness in his epigastric region. Bowel sounds were present and sounded normal. There was no meningism or clouded mental state.

Clinical comment

Bearing in mind the possible diagnoses and the findings elicited so far, the following investigations could be justified:

- Chest X-ray: looking for consolidation
- Full blood count: assessing the white cell count as a response to inflammation
- U&Es: assessing electrolyte status and renal function, both of which could be abnormal given his dehydration and possible metabolic acidosis
- Lipase: pancreatitis could be a possibility, given epigastric tenderness and abnormal vital signs
- Blood cultures: to identify a cause of sepsis.

The arterial blood gas results become available (see Table 6.1 below).

Table 6.1 Arterial blood gas results

Result	Level	Normal range
FIO_2	0.58	As calculated above
pH	7.15	7.35–7.45
pCO_2	12	35–45 mmHg
pO_2	291	80–100 mmHg
HCO_3	11	22–32 mmol/L
Base excess	−9.2	−3 – +3
Blood glucose	25	< 7.7 mmol/L
Lactate	3.2	< 0.8 mmol/L
Na	127	135–145 mmol/L
K	6.2	3.5–4.5 mmol/L

Clinical question 3

Comment upon the ABG. What is the diagnosis? Consider how you would present this patient to a senior colleague.

The intern studies the blood gas, noting the significant abnormalities that are present. However, there are multiple components to the blood gas and she considers them carefully before presenting her findings to the consultant.

'John is a 24-year-old man who presents with diabetic ketoacidosis with a blood sugar level (BSL) of 25. This is his first presentation with diabetes, and he's usually well and in good health. He's been unwell for 4 days with symptoms of a respiratory tract infection, but in the past 2 days he's had polyuria and polydipsia and features of significant dehydration. He collapsed today on standing, and he's tachycardic and hypotensive. I've started a bag of normal saline, and his arterial blood gas shows a decompensated metabolic acidosis. I've requested a series of bloods and I'm waiting on a chest X-ray to see if there are any features of pneumonia that may have precipitated this event. I'm going to give a 6 unit bolus of insulin and then start an insulin infusion at 0.1 units per kg per hour, as per the hospital protocol.'

The consultant looks at the blood gas result.

'What will you do about his potassium? It's quite high...'

The intern looks at the gas again.

'Yes, it is ... we can do an ECG and see if there are any changes; I'll get some calcium gluconate ready and when we start the insulin infusion that should bring the level down.'

The consultant nods.

'Good. We'll then have to monitor the potassium very closely—his total body potassium levels are likely to be low and will plummet further once we start therapy, and we'll need to provide replacement once the level falls below 5 mmol/L. Be careful with the fluid replacement—we don't want to replace too much too quickly.'

The intern returns to the patient to start the therapy and to discuss his diagnosis with him.

Physiology comment

There are two types of diabetes: type 1 and type 2. Patients with type 1 diabetes, or insulin-dependent diabetes mellitus (IDDM), can develop a condition known as diabetic ketoacidosis (DKA). DKA is a metabolic state caused by a diabetes-induced insulin deficit that results in hyperglycaemia and elevated plasma ketone bodies (> 5 mmol/L). Insulin is an anabolic hormone and a deficit results in abnormal metabolism that eventually leads to the mobilisation of lipids. As we will see later, frequent urination, rapid deep respirations, nausea and vomiting are all signs of a progressing insulin deficit.

A lack of insulin restricts the movement of glucose across the cell membrane, forcing the body to rely on other food classes for energy production. Utilisation of lipids (and to a lesser extent proteins) instead of glucose as an energy substrate at the cellular level leads to elevated levels of fatty acids and their metabolic by-products appearing in the blood. These metabolites are known as ketone bodies or ketoacids, and consist of acetone and two organic acids (beta-hydroxybutyric acid and acetoacetic acid). The acetone breath often exhibited by patients with DKA is caused by the elevated levels of these metabolites in the pulmonary capillary blood tainting the alveolar gas. The rapid deep panting also frequently observed is caused by the body attempting to compensate for a metabolic acidosis caused by the accumulation of the ketoacids. Increasing the rate and depth of breathing and therefore blowing off CO_2 will go some way to compensate for the developing metabolic acidosis.

Patients with diabetic ketoacidosis typically have a fluid deficit of 3–5 L upon admission. This level of volume loss is obviously significant and the likely development of hypovolaemic shock should always be at the forefront of the treating physician's mind. Patients presenting with DKA also tend to be deficient of Na and K, because of excessive losses in the urine. An osmotic diuresis in DKA is caused by an elevated glucose loading in the nephrons of the kidney. The transport maximum of each nephron is overwhelmed by the unusually high glucose load, and glucose begins to enter the latter parts of the nephron instead of being fully reabsorbed by the end of the proximal tubule. Glucose in the distal parts of the nephron tubule exerts an osmotic force that causes the retention of water and associated ions in the collecting duct filtrate. This eventually leads to a pronounced osmotic diuresis and therefore frequent urination, one of the signs of diabetes.

Serum values of electrolytes may be misleading in DKA as water is lost along with electrolytes. Measured electrolyte concentrations may possibly be elevated even though there is an overall total body deficit. This is not because total body electrolyte has increased, but because relatively more water has been lost than the electrolyte. Care must always be taken to interpret electrolyte values along with an assessment of body fluid status and to be aware that ingestion of large volumes of pure water may also influence electrolyte readings. In addition, Na levels may be factitiously low due to the high blood glucose level (BGL) interfering with the accuracy of the Na measurement.

Clinical comment

The intern made an excellent presentation in that the diagnosis was mentioned early, unambiguously and prominently. In a desire to be thorough, too often important aspects of the history and examination seem to be hidden amid a large amount of important but not immediately relevant information. Junior staff must learn to assemble information, prioritise relevant features, and present them to senior staff in a time-critical manner.

In this instance, the high glucose in the presence of a metabolic acidosis confirms the diagnosis of diabetic ketoacidosis. Aggressive treatment is indicated, with careful attention being paid to hydration status and electrolyte balance. Different hospitals have different protocols for managing this condition, so detailed management will not be discussed here. However, close attention must always be paid to the potassium level: an initially high result will rapidly normalise and then the level will become dangerously low once potassium starts moving back into the cells as a result of the correction of the acidosis and the start of insulin therapy. The patient is likely to be depleted of potassium as a result of the osmotic diuresis caused by the hyperglycaemic state preceding the ketoacidosis. Hence, potassium is usually replaced once the potassium level falls below 5 mmol/L.

Similarly, once the glucose level falls below 14 mmol/L the intravenous fluid is usually changed to 5% dextrose so that exogenous glucose can be provided and hypoglycaemia does not occur.

Physiology comment

Appropriate management of acute DKA aims to normalise any changes to the underlying physiology that have been brought about by the altered metabolic state. This includes:

- Restoration of intravascular volume loss
- Control of blood glucose by using exogenous insulin
- Replacement of any K losses

- Correction of acid–base disturbance if severe
- Replacement of phosphate if significant.

An infusion of normal saline quickly re-expands the vascular space, correcting any life-threatening hypovolaemia. A treating physician should be aware that K levels may drop (leading to a life-threatening hypokalaemia) as a secondary to any insulin therapy, and therefore early K replacement may be warranted. Correction of an underlying acid–base disturbance with bicarbonate therapy is controversial, as bicarbonate therapy may cause paradoxical CNS acidosis and the rapid correction of acidosis caused by bicarbonate may also result in hypokalaemia. Bicarbonate may be of use in selected patients with a pH under 6.9. Therapy is directed at correcting the underlying cause of the acidosis itself, rather than normalising the blood gas values.

Epilogue

John's chest X-ray was normal and he was diagnosed with bronchitis; no specific treatment was required for this condition. He was admitted to the intensive care unit for continued fluid resuscitation and close monitoring. An arterial line was inserted into his left radial artery so that repeated blood gas sampling could be performed. His potassium quickly dropped and required replacement. After 24 hours his glucose normalised, his acidosis had been corrected, and he was changed from an insulin infusion to a subcutaneous insulin regime. He was visited by the hospital's diabetic educator who gave him advice about the necessary changes to his life now that he was diagnosed as a type 1 diabetic.

Tips

- A bedside blood glucose level performed earlier would have enabled an earlier diagnosis to be made in this case.
- Finding the precipitant of the acute presentation is important—simply diagnosing the ketoacidosis is not sufficient.
- Venous blood gas values are as helpful as arterial blood gas values in assessing acid–base status and in guiding therapy, and obtaining the sample is significantly less painful for the patient.
- Careful and regular attention to potassium levels is paramount.

References and further reading

1 Bateman, N.T. & Leach, R.M. ABC of oxygen: Acute oxygen therapy. *BMJ* 1998; 317: 798–801.
2 Charfen, M.A. & Fernández-Frackelton, M. Diabetic ketoacidosis. *Emerg Med Clin N Am* Aug 2005; 23 (3): 609–28.
3 Hardern, R.D. & Quinn, N.D. Emergency management of diabetic ketoacidosis in adults, *Emerg Med J* 2003; 20: 210–13.
4 Solá, E., Garzón, S., García-Torres, S. et al. Management of diabetic ketoacidosis in a teaching hospital, *Acta Diabetol* 2006; 43: 127–30, doi: 10.1007/s00592-006-0227-1
5 Wallace, T.M. & Matthews, D.R. Recent advances in the monitoring and management of diabetic ketoacidosis. *Q J Med* 2004; 97: 773–80, doi: 10.1093/qjmed/hch132

Case review

Basic science questions

1 The ECF volume deficit seen in patients with DKA is caused primarily by which of the following?

   A Reduced fluid intake
   B Reduced production of metabolic water
   C Increased losses through the gastrointestinal tract
   D Increased renal losses
   E Increased evaporated losses

2 The acetone breath often exhibited by patients with DKA is caused by the accumulation of which metabolite?

   A Insulin
   B Glucagon
   C Keto acids
   D Urea
   E Creatinine

3 The reabsorption of glucose takes place in which region(s) of the nephron?

   A Proximal tubule only
   B Distal tubule only
   C Loop of Henle only
   D All tubular segments
   E Proximal tubule and collecting ducts

Clinical questions

1 Match the following blood gas results with the most fitting descriptions:

A pH 7.13 pO_2 85 pCO_2 13 HCO_3 12
B pH 7.23 pO_2 58 pCO_2 83 HCO_3 32
C pH 7.53 pO_2 62 pCO_2 13 HCO_3 24
D pH 7.49 pO_2 85 pCO_2 39 HCO_3 38

   (i)   Metabolic acidosis
   (ii) Metabolic alkalosis
   (iii) Respiratory acidosis
   (iv) Respiratory alkalosis

2 Which of the following are not clinical features of diabetic ketoacidosis?

A Polydipsia
B Altered mental state
C Hypoventilation
D Dehydration
E Normal–high blood glucose level

3 Which of the following fluids should not be used in the management of DKA?

A 0.9% normal saline
B 5% dextrose
C 0.9% normal saline with 30 mmol/L KCl
D 2.7% hypertonic saline
E Hartmann's solution

Case 7
Mr Wallis couldn't breathe …

Mr Wallis was a pleasant elderly fellow who'd been in reasonable health most of his life, but lately he'd been getting increasingly breathless and unable to do what he'd like to do. His GP had started him on some tablets for it, but today he was suddenly feeling a lot worse. He's puffing away when you see him …

Clinical learning objectives

- Know how to assess and manage a patient presenting with breathlessness.
- Be able to use pathological and radiological investigations rationally to investigate breathless patients.
- Know the life-threatening causes of breathlessness and their emergency management.
- Understand the role of multidisciplinary teams and the importance of clinical guidelines and pathways to optimise patient care in chronic disease.

Physiology learning objectives

- Describe the two main categories of pulmonary oedema.
- Outline how and why congestive cardiac failure (CCF) is associated with atrial fibrillation.
- Understand how CCF can lead to inappropriate reabsorption of salt and water by the kidneys.
- Describe the factors controlling β-type natriuretic factor release.
- Understand the role of potassium in normal body function.
- Define hypokalaemia and understand how it may be caused.
- Explain the physiological basis for the treatment of hypokalaemia.
- Describe how and why hypokalaemia alters the ECG.

Timeline

10:30	Mr Wallis presents to emergency complaining of breathlessness; triaged category 3 as 'increasing breathlessness, worse today'.
10:50	Medical assessment and initial treatment begins.
11:30	Not improving; additional therapy commenced.
12:15	Results available; referred for admission.

Clinical presentation

Joe Wallis was a healthy 77-year-old who lived at home alone and was in excellent health, apart from some mild hypertension. He'd started feeling breathless when walking down to the local shops for at least a few weeks, and his GP had started him on 'a fluid tablet' to assist. He'd been feeling a little better (despite peeing so much after taking the tablets), but for the past 2 days he'd had a dry cough and a fever. This morning he couldn't catch his breath no matter what he did, so he rang his neighbour and asked him to drive him to the local hospital.

10:30 hours

Joe's neighbour dropped him off in front of the emergency department. He shuffled over to the triage desk and explained his problem to the triage nurse. Recognising that he was out of breath and looked unwell, she called the orderly and arranged for him to be moved straight in onto a bed in a cubicle. He was briefly assessed as being breathless, and was assigned a triage category 3. He was placed on to a bed and moved into a cubicle. Monitoring equipment is attached and his vital signs are recorded as follows:

- PR   110 irregular
- BP   180/85
- RR   24
- Temp   37.5°C
- SpO_2 94% RA

10:50 hours

The resident logs his name against Joe's on the computer and introduces himself. As he approaches the bed, the nurse is in the process of recording an ECG.

Clinical question 1

Describe your initial actions upon meeting Joe. What could be going on? How will you commence your assessment?

Clinical comment

Joe has self-presented to the triage desk, so it is essential that triage staff recognise early that he is acutely unwell. Overcrowding and access block mean it may not always be possible for stable patients to move directly in to the treatment area, but, when acutely unwell patients present, every possible effort is made to accommodate them and to begin treatment as soon as possible. Innovative methods of improving patient flow all the way along the patient journey pathway are being trialled and introduced into hospitals.

Initial actions are based around the well-described standardised approach to the assessment and management of the patient with an undifferentiated illness. Assessment of the airway, breathing and circulation is an important first step. In Joe's case, he is talking, so it can be assumed his airway is patent. He is breathless, so supplemental oxygen can assist the patient without having to have a specific diagnosis. His circulation can be assessed by the objective measurements of pulse and blood pressure, but these must be assessed in the context of his conscious state and peripheral perfusion in order to obtain an accurate full picture.

There are many causes of acute breathlessness. The following diagnoses could be considered as the resident assesses Joe:

- Chest infection: bronchitis, or pneumonia
- Cardiovascular causes: pulmonary oedema and congestive cardiac failure, myocardial ischaemia, dysrhythmias, or pulmonary embolus
- Exacerbation of chronic obstructive pulmonary disease, or asthma
- Anaemia
- Malignancy: lung, or metastatic disease.

With these possibilities in mind it is important to take a directed history. This is essentially testing hypotheses. A number of possibilities can readily be ruled out by history and examination. It is important to prioritise the approach and immediately consider life-threatening conditions that require a time-critical response. The emergency department assessment of a patient such as Joe means more than just making a diagnosis—it also involves stratifying risk and starting therapy, often without all the information being available. All of this must be done in the context of a busy department, and with the understanding that even a small delay at each stage will prolong his length of stay within the department and impact upon both his and other patients' care.

The resident medical officer (RMO) reviews the observations, and begins his assessment by introducing himself to Joe as he finishes having his ECG.

RMO: 'Hi Joe, my name's Peter. What's brought you here today?'

Joe: 'I can't breathe ... it got worse this morning. I could hardly sleep last night ...'

RMO: 'How long has this been a problem?'

Joe: 'It's been getting worse for weeks, now. My doctor started me on a tablet and that has helped a little, but the past 2 days I seem to be getting a cold and it's knocked me flat.'

RMO: 'Any coughs or fevers?'

Joe: 'Just a dry cough, which is worse in the evening.'

Clinical comment

At this point the RMO's questioning is heading down an infective path. It is important to consider infection, but it's essential to not get side-tracked. The nurse hands him the following ECG for review (see Figure 7.1 below).

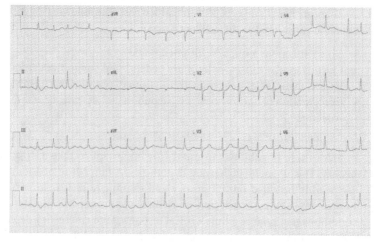

Figure 7.1 Joe's 12-lead ECG

Clinical question 2

Interpret the ECG and describe it. What questions should you be asking now?

Clinical comment

The ECG is irregularly irregular with no readily identifiable P waves. This is atrial fibrillation, which is an important precipitant for decompensated congestive cardiac failure. Just as the treating team must actively look for the precipitant underlying the cardiac failure, they must also consider the underlying cause of the atrial fibrillation.

The focus of the assessment should now shift towards investigating a possible cardiac cause for Joe's symptoms.

Physiology comment

Pulmonary oedema is the abnormal accumulation of fluid in the interstitial spaces surrounding alveoli, with possible fluid exudation into alveolar air space. Pulmonary oedema can usefully be considered under 2 main categories, based upon the physiological cause:

1 High pressure, hydrostatic and cardiogenic refer to an elevated pulmonary capillary hydrostatic cause
2 Low pressure, high permeability and non-cardiogenic refer to conditions where permeability is elevated.

Atrial fibrillation

Atrial fibrillation (AF) is an irregular rhythm generated by disorganised atrial depolarisation, with random conduction of some impulses through the atrio-ventricular (AV) junction to the ventricles. Chronic CCF is associated with atrial fibrillation because CCF-induced atrial deformation stretches the atria, leading to enhanced automaticity and multiple re-entry circuits. The increased resistance at the AV node normally blocks most atrial impulses, but the ventricular rate is often in excess of 200 bpm. The faster the ventricular rate the greater the decrease in cardiac output, because both stroke volume and cardiac output are reduced. The ECG shows an irregular rhythm with P waves replaced with a characteristic wavy baseline (F waves). The QRS complex will be normal unless additional conduction abnormalities occur downstream of the AV node.

Peter the RMO looks at Joe: 'Your ECG shows you're in an irregular heart beat. Has this been a problem for you for long?'
Joe replies 'No—never heard of that as a problem …'
Peter inserts an IV cannula and draws blood for analysis. He obtains the following history, which he later records in the notes:

- Seventy-seven year old male, Hx hypertension; lives alone independently; and an ex-smoker
- Meds—thiazide diuretic; recently started on ?frusemide (pt not sure)
- Two months of orthopnoea and paroxysmal nocturnal dyspnoea
- Occasional ankle swelling; and breathless after 20 metres of walking on flat ground
- Denies chest pain or discomfort
- Occasionally aware of palpitations
- No weight loss; and no haemoptysis—thinks he has gained weight in the past 2 weeks
- No recent immobilisation or operations.

Before Peter conducts a full physical examination, he listens to Joe's chest. He hears coarse crackles at both bases.

Clinical question 3

(a) Given the history and the brief examination, what is the most likely diagnosis?
(b) Is there any therapy you would start now, or would you complete the examination and await investigations?

Clinical comment

It appears that Joe is suffering from decompensated congestive heart failure, as indicated by the orthopnoea, the paroxysmal nocturnal dyspnoea, and the clinical finding of crackles on his chest. He is not critically unwell and is not in acute pulmonary oedema, either of which would require a markedly different approach to the management of the pathophysiology and resuscitation. It is not enough to make a diagnosis of congestive heart failure alone, however—the precipitant must be identified. Joe has long-standing hypertension, and he is in atrial fibrillation—two significant causes of heart failure in this community. These may be long-standing, and it's possible that the recent respiratory tract infection has more acutely worsened his condition. There is much to investigate and sort out, but at this point hastening Joe's treatment and flow through the department is worthwhile—a good start is to administer additional diuretic therapy and send appropriate blood tests.

Physiology comment

In the later stages of CCF the renal system inappropriately reabsorbs both salt and water. This leads to an expansion of the extracellular fluid volume, further worsening any central and peripheral oedema already present. The renal system is stimulated to reabsorb salt and water by the reduction in blood pressure brought about by the cardiac failure. The lowered blood pressure is sensed by both intrarenal (afferent arteriolar and macula densa) pressure/flow receptors and extrarenal (cardiovascular baroreceptors) receptors that bring about activation of the renin–angiotensin–aldosterone system.

The renal system has no way of responding directly to changes in extracellular fluid (ECF) volume, and instead relies upon an indirect measure of blood pressure to alter salt and water balance. Under normal conditions, ECF volume and total body sodium decrease and increase in step with blood pressure. In CCF, however, the link between increasing ECF volume (preload) and increasing blood pressure is lost because the heart is failing. Therefore the blood pressure remains low even though the ECF volume is progressively increasing (and blood pressure may even fall if the myocardium is overstretched), and the kidney expands the ECF volume even further via a reflex mechanism.

Factors controlling β-type natriuretic factor release

Cells in the cardiac atria secrete a peptide hormone called β-type natriuretic protein (BNP) when the atria are overstretched (as seen during ECF volume expansion) in CCF. β-type natriuretic factor acts to inhibit sodium reabsorption by the nephron directly or indirectly, and therefore to some degree offsets the almost total reabsorption of sodium that occurs in CCF.

Peter writes a drug order for 40 mg of intravenous frusemide, and requests the blood tests FBC, U&E, LFT, troponin, BNP, and Ca, Mg & PO_4. He also submits a request for a chest X-ray.

Peter proceeds to fully examine Joe and records the following findings:

- Breathless, can only talk in short sentences
- PR   110 AF
- BP   180/85
- RR   24
- SpO$_2$ 98% 6 L O$_2$/min
- JVP not seen
- Apex beat displaced to left anterior axillary line
- HS dual + 3rd heart sound
- Mild pitting oedema to mid lower legs
- Chest:

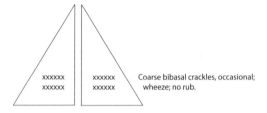

Coarse bibasal crackles, occasional; wheeze; no rub.

- Abdo: soft, non-tender.

Peter collects his thoughts and presents his findings to the consultant.

11:30 hours

Joe is still feeling breathless, despite having passed approximately 500 mL of urine after receiving the diuretic. His heart is still racing at up to 120 beats per minute, and he is feeling tired. He has had his chest X-ray (see Figure 7.2 overleaf). The pathology lab rings to notify that one of his tests is abnormal: he has a K of 2.6 mmol/L.

Physiology comment

Potassium is involved in cell growth and division, the establishment and maintenance of membrane potentials, regulating intracellular volume, and hydrogen balance. As the kidney is the major organ responsible for regulating loss or output of potassium from the body, evaluating potassium status is very important from a clinical perspective. Even slight deviations from the normal range of 3.5–5.5 mmol/L can have serious consequences, such as cardiac arrhythmias.

The concentration of potassium is high within the cells (150 mmol/L), with a total body amount of close to 3500 mmol. The low extracellular concentration of approximately 4.5 mmol/L is maintained by potassium shifting between the extracellular and intracellular spaces. This movement is regulated or influenced by factors such as insulin, catecholamines, pH and aldosterone, and is termed 'internal balance'. External balance is regulated by input (diet) and output (renal and gastrointestinal losses). The renal system is the more important of these two output routes, and is responsible for excreting 95% of the typical daily load.

Hypokalaemia can be defined as a plasma concentration of less than 3.5 mmol/L. It can be caused by reduced input, redistribution between body fluid compartments, or increased losses. Dietary causes for hypokalaemia are relatively rare, as potassium is found in many common foodstuffs. The movement of potassium from the ECF into the ICF is more common, and can be caused by factors such as insulin therapy, metabolic alkalosis, and administration of salbutamol. Increased output is also a common cause of hypokalaemia, with vomiting, diarrhoea and laxative abuse all contributing to increased loss from the body. Hyperaldosteronism, whether primary or secondary, will lead to increased renal excretion, as will administration of diuretics. In this case the administration of a loop diuretic that acts directly to block potassium reabsorption in the Loop of Henle, and indirectly increased potassium secretion from the late distal tubule and collecting ducts, has most likely led to the development of the hypokalaemia.

Close monitoring of the plasma potassium levels of patients at risk is important, as hypokalaemia can quickly lead to the development of life-threatening cardiac dysrhythmias. Treatment of hypokalaemia is based on the progressive replacement of potassium, either orally or intravenously. Correction of any co-existing alkalosis will often be enough to address any hypokalaemia present, as the normalisation of pH acts to shift potassium from the ICF into the ECF. Obviously care needs to be taken to monitor potassium levels closely throughout this process. If loss of potassium is suspected as a possible cause of the hypokalaemia, steps should be taken to remove the underlying cause if possible.

The ECG typically displays a typical pattern of flattened T waves, a prolonged QT interval, and the appearance of U waves. The changes to the ECG are brought about by the reduction in the resting membrane potential of cardiac cells that is caused by the low ECF potassium. This hyperpolarises the cell membrane (resting membrane potential becomes further away from the threshold potential), making the cells less excitable.

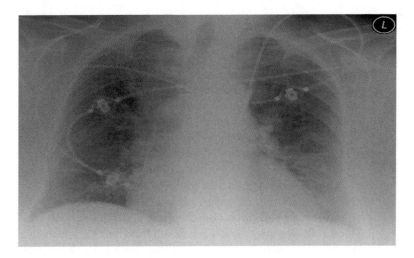

Figure 7.2 Joe's chest X-ray

Clinical question 4

What will you do now?

Clinical comment

A number of therapies need to be considered. Joe has a rapid ventricular rate that will be impairing his cardiac output; so rate control with an agent that is not a negative inotrope would be ideal—digoxin is useful for this purpose. It is also important to optimise his electrolyte balance—the low potassium, likely to have been precipitated by the dual action of a thiazide and a loop diuretic, could explain his frequent ectopic beats and be a contributor to his worsening cardiac function. Correcting the hypokalaemia is a priority. Using oral agents in the first instance is recommended, as intravenous potassium needs to be diluted significantly, which would require a large volume of fluid to be administered—and this would be counterproductive in this case.

It is likely that a degree of cardiac ischaemia is present; so pre-emptive treatment with aspirin and an anticoagulant (which reduces the risk of thromboembolic disease developing in patients with atrial fibrillation) must be considered. The chest X-ray is consistent with heart failure, with cardiomegaly and upper lobe vascular redistribution.

12:15 hours

After discussion with the consultant, the resident writes up the medication (see Table 7.1 below).

Table 7.1 Medication

Date/time	Drug	Dose	Route	Signed
27/12 12:15	Digoxin	500 µg	IV	Peter R
	Aspirin	300 mg	Oral	Peter R
	Enoxaparin	80 mg	Subcutaneous	Peter R
	Chlorvescent	2 tablets	Oral	Peter R
	Slow K	2 tablets	Oral	Peter R
	MgCl	10 mmol	IV slow push	Peter R

The rest of the blood tests become available (see Table 7.2 below).

Table 7.2 Blood test results

Result	Level	Normal range
Biochemistry		
Na	133	135–145 mmol/L
K	2.6	3.5–4.5 mmol/L
Cl	96	95–110 mmol/L
HCO_3	25	22–32 mmol/L
Urea	7.8	3.0–8.0 mmol/L
Creatinine	0.109	< 0.110 mmol/L
Anion gap	13	8–16 mmol/L
Troponin	0.05	< 0.03 mmol/L
BNP	1456 pg/mL	< 100 makes HF less likely
Haematology		
Hb	114	130–180 g/L
WCC	11.3	$4.0–11.0 \times 10^9$/L
Neutrophils	9.4	–
Platelets	167	$150–400 \times 10^9$/L

The resident rings the medical registrar to make his referral:

'Hello, I'm ringing to refer Mr Wallis, a 77-year-old male who lives alone independently and presents with decompensated heart failure. He has a history of hypertension treated with a thiazide diuretic, and he takes ibuprofen for arthritis in his knees. He's had symptoms of orthopnoea and breathlessness on mild exertion for a few weeks now, and has partially responded to oral frusemide. He's been acutely unwell for the past 2 days, with symptoms of bronchitis. This morning he was acutely breathless, he's in AF with a rate of up to 120, and he's hypertensive. He's got pitting oedema in his ankles and crackles in his lower left and right chest. His ECG shows AF and his potassium is low at 2.6. His BNP is high and he has a negative troponin.

'I've done a few things: he's had 40 mg of IV frusemide, as well as 500 μg of IV digoxin for rate control; he's had 300 mg of aspirin and 80 mg of Enoxaparin for presumed cardiac ischaemia; and I've started to correct his low potassium with oral potassium and IV magnesium. He needs to be admitted to be stabilised, have an echocardiogram, and commence an ACE inhibitor and other drugs as indicated. I've suggested he stop taking his non-steroidal anti-inflammatory drug (NSAID) and use paracetamol instead, and I've started him on the heart failure pathway.'

Clinical comment

A short and to-the-point referral is essential, whether to the consultant in the emergency department or to the admitting team. Referring doctors need to prioritise important points and make it clear what the diagnosis is, what they've done, and what it actually is that they're asking for (e.g. advice, admission, or an urgent outpatient appointment). The increasing use of clinical pathways is an important way to improve safety and quality and to bridge the gap between evidence and practice.

β-type natriuretic protein is increasingly being used to improve the diagnosis of heart failure. It can be used to help guide therapy in breathless patients where the diagnosis is not immediately clear, and it is being used to improve risk stratification in patients with other forms of heart disease.

The National Institute of Clinical Studies has focused on improving the diagnosis and management of heart failure as one of its key projects—an important goal, given the rising prevalence of heart failure in an ageing population with large numbers of risk factors for cardiovascular disease.

Emergency departments provide an essential link in the care of these patients, and in identifying patients at risk of developing heart failure. Optimising medication is a key part of such a strategy; for example, as in Joe's case, NSAIDS promote fluid retention and can worsen heart failure, and should not be used where a better alternative (such as paracetamol) exists.

Epilogue

Joe was admitted to a medical ward and commenced on anti-failure therapy comprising of an ACE inhibitor and frusemide. An echocardiogram revealed hypertrophic changes of the myocardium consistent with long-standing hypertension, but no valvular disease. Rate control of his AF was achieved with digoxin, and he was commenced on oral anticoagulant therapy with warfarin for thromboembolic prophylaxis. His potassium level was soon corrected and he remained on potassium replacement therapy to optimise his cardiac function.

A heart failure nurse practitioner visits him regularly at home, and works closely with his general practitioner to monitor his cardiac function and to pre-empt any exacerbations of his condition.

Tips

- Positioning patients in an upright position and administering oxygen is a useful starting point for breathless patients, regardless of the cause.
- Obtaining an up-to-date list of the patient's medication can help optimise therapy and identify precipitants.
- Making a diagnosis of heart failure is not sufficient: the precipitant must be identified and treated.
- Optimising electrolyte balance can improve heart function.

References and further reading

1 Abhayaratna, W.P., Smith, W.T., Becker, N.G. et al. Prevalence of heart failure and systolic ventricular dysfunction in older Australians: The Canberra Heart Study, *MJA* 2006; 184: 151–4.
2 Chircop, R. & Jelinek, G.A. β-type natriuretic peptide in the diagnosis of heart failure in the emergency department. *Emerg Med Australas* 2006; 18: 170–9.

3 Harrison, A. & Amundson, S. Evaluation and management of the acutely dyspneic patient: The role of biomarkers. *Am J Emerg Med* 2005; 23: 371–8.
4 National Heart Foundation of Australia and the Cardiac Society of Australia and New Zealand (Chronic Heart Failure Guidelines Expert Writing Panel), *Guidelines for the prevention, detection and management of chronic heart failure in Australia, 2006*, National Heart Foundation, Melbourne, 2007.
5 National Institute of Clinical Studies. Heart failure forum 2004: Improving outcomes in chronic care. Report. NICS, Melbourne, 2004.
6 Sosnowski, M.A. Lack of effect of opiates in the treatment of acute cardiogenic pulmonary oedema. *Emerg Med Australas* 2008; 20: 384–90.

Case review

Basic science questions

1 In later stages of CCF:
   A Sodium reabsorption by the kidney is increased
   B Sodium reabsorption by the kidney is reduced
   C The ECF volume is reduced
   D The ICF volume is reduced
   E Pulmonary capillary pressures are often reduced
2 Hypokalaemia can be defined as a plasma concentration of less than what value?
   A 10 mmol/L
   B 15 mmol/L
   C 0.5 mmol/L
   D 3.5 mmol/L
   E 6 mmol/L
3 The typical ECG pattern associated with hypokalaemia reveals:
   A A normal sinus rhythm
   B U waves and flattened T waves
   C Shortened QT intervals
   D No U waves and an extended PR interval
   E An inverted QRS complex

Clinical questions

1 Which of the following drugs should be avoided in heart failure?
   A Digoxin
   B Carvedilol
   C Verapamil
   D ACE inhibitors
   E Aspirin

2 Which of the following conditions can exacerbate heart failure?
   A Chest infection
   B Atrial fibrillation
   C Acute coronary syndrome
   D Hypertensive crisis
   E All of the above
3 Which of the following therapies would be the least helpful in managing acute decompensated heart failure?
   A Continuous positive airway pressure (CPAP)
   B Frusemide
   C Intravenous glyceryl trinitrate
   D 100% oxygen
   E 2 mg increments of intravenous morphine

Case 8
Mark had a pain in his belly that wouldn't go away...

Mark was a 54-year-old male who'd felt 'off' for a few days but now had worsening upper abdominal pain. He says it's his ulcer playing up but you're worried it could be more than that ...

Clinical learning objectives

- Know the important causes of upper abdominal pain and how they present.
- Be able to use pathological and radiological investigations to conduct a rational investigation of the causes of upper abdominal pain in a time-effective manner.
- Understand how to approach a patient with abdominal pain, regardless of the cause.
- Be able to apply clinical scoring systems to patients for the purposes of prognosis and disposition.

Physiological learning objectives

- Define pancreatitis and describe what factors can lead to its development.
- Describe the physiological consequences of pancreatitis.
- Define anion gap and explain why it is elevated in this case.
- Describe the mechanism by which pancreatitis can lead to the development of a metabolic acidosis and hypocalcaemia.
- Define the term 'base excess' and explain how and why it is elevated in this case.

Timeline

09:30	Pain in abdomen worsening, Mark proceeds to hospital.
10:10	Self-presents to emergency department; triaged category 3; moved into cubicle and observations taken.
10:27	Seen by the intern, assessment and initial treatment begins.
10:50	Presents findings to the consultant, confirms plan.
11:35	X-ray available for viewing.
12:15	Initial results available; definitive management arranged.

Clinical presentation

Mark was a tiler in his mid-50s who worked six days a week. He had no previous medical conditions to speak of. He'd been getting intermittent abdominal pains for the past 12 months that he'd self-diagnosed as an ulcer, and he would take an antacid to relieve the symptoms. He hadn't seen his doctor about it as the pain would usually settle after 1 or 2 days.

Today, though, was different. The pain was more intense: a deep burning, radiating through to his back. It wouldn't settle despite increasing doses of antacids, and he just couldn't get comfortable. He hadn't slept at all overnight and called in sick to work. By 9:30 in the morning he couldn't stand it any longer and he asked his wife to drive him to the hospital. She dropped him off at the emergency department, where he was assisted into a wheelchair and presented to the triage nurse.

10:10 hours

He is assessed by the triage nurse, who notes how uncomfortable he looks: he is pale, clutching his abdomen, and is unwilling to walk. A brief history is obtained and he is assigned a triage category of 3 with a description of 'upper abdominal pain?ulcer'. A bed within a cubicle is available and with the assistance of an orderly he is moved into the department and on to the bed.

The nurse assigned to that cubicle introduces himself and takes a focused history. He also takes and records vital signs:

- Fifty-four year old male, 2 days of abdominal pain; epigastric pain radiating to back; previous history of ulcer; meds—nil and allergies—nil
- PR   106 bpm
- BP   120/85

- RR   20
- Temp   37.4°C
- SpO$_2$ 97% RA
- Looks uncomfortable, pain 7/10

With the vitals signs taken, Mark awaits assessment by a doctor.

Clinical question 1

What additional actions could the nurse or other staff take to improve Mark's time to treatment?

10:27 hours

Allison, the intern, logs her name against Mark's name on the departmental computer, and enters the cubicle. She reads the nursing notes and prepares to start her assessment.

She sees Mark lying on the bed, sweating profusely, clutching his abdomen. Recognising that he is in significant pain, she offers him some pain relief prior to any other action. He nods vigorously, and Allison inserts an 18 gauge intravenous cannula into the dorsum of his right hand. At the same time blood is collected and the cannula is secured. Allison turns to the nurse:

'Could you please draw up 10 mg of morphine and titrate it in 5 mg boluses to make him comfortable? I've also written up 10 mg of metoclopramide as well as 1 L of normal saline to be given over an hour.'

She turns to Mark and begins her assessment.

Clinical question 2

(a) What possible diagnoses are you considering based upon the basic information provided so far?
(b) What important questions will you need to ask to make a diagnosis?

Clinical comment

Early assessment and pain relief can not only improve the time to analgesia, which is both humane and an important quality indicator, but can hasten diagnosis and shorten departmental length of stay. By itself this may not seem significant, but with access block and emergency department overcrowding increasingly impacting upon patient care, it can make a difference to the care of the patient population as a whole. Many departments have introduced 'fast track' systems to improve flows and processes. These facilitate teamwork, but challenge traditional perceptions of doctor, nursing and other professionals' roles within the team. Nursing staff can ably perform procedures once considered the domain of medical staff: intravenous cannulation, administration of analgesia, taking histories, ordering investigations, and performing selected procedures. In this instance, early cannulation and providing intravenous analgesia would have shortened the time to making a diagnosis and arranging disposition.

There are a number of causes for acute epigastric pain, each with particular characteristics and methods of investigation. Treating doctors need to consider peptic ulcer disease and its complications, pancreatitis, hepatobiliary disease, inferior myocardial ischaemia, aortic dissection, and pulmonary causes such as lower lobe pneumonia. Important questions to ask would include:

- What is the nature of the pain: sudden onset, colicky, burning, or constant in nature?
- Is there was a confirmed history of ulcers (remember that only Mark has called his condition an 'ulcer')?
- Is there any:
  - History of indigestion?
  - Recent weight loss or pain during or after eating?
  - Haematemesis or melaena?
  - Jaundice or history suggesting liver disease?
  - Use of non-steroidal anti-inflammatory drugs (NSAIDs)?
  - History of alcohol use (specifically quantify the amount)?
  - Chest pain or symptoms associated with myocardial ischaemia?
  - Coughs, colds or fevers suggestive of a respiratory tract infection?

Consideration of these symptoms can help staff focus in on a diagnosis prior to examination or ordering investigations.

Allison takes a history and writes her notes in point form as she talks with Mark:

- Two days of intermittent, then constant upper abdominal pain radiating through to back
- Off food, and poor oral intake; feels nauseated; and no vomiting or haematemesis

- Bowels opened 2 days ago, none since, and is passing flatus
- Feels hot, but no documented fever
- No chest pain
- No history of jaundice
- Past history: nil significant; intermittent abdominal pain past 1–2 years, never investigated
- Social history: is married to Joan, works as a tiler and has 2 adult children; smokes 15 cigarettes per day × 40 years; and drinks ~6 standard drinks per day (beer).

His pain has eased a great deal with 10 mg of morphine, and Allison starts to examine him. She records her findings as follows:

- Looks pale and dehydrated with dry mucous membranes
- No jaundice
- Occasional spider naevi around left and right shoulders
- PR 110 bpm   BP 120/70   RR 24   Temp 37.4°C
- HS × 2 nil added
- Chest: clear.

No liver palpable   Tip of spleen palpable

////////
////////   ← Tender+++ with guarding

No AAA

No hernias

BS scant

No ascites

Kidneys not palpable

PR examination: no blood, no masses, prostate normal

Clinical question 3

(a) Based upon this information, what is your likely diagnosis?
(b) How will you test this hypothesis? What investigations will you perform?
(c) How will you manage Mark until the results come back?
(d) Tie these questions together by considering how you would present Mark as a patient to the consultant.

Allison is thinking about her plan of action as she writes her notes. She sends the bloods to pathology and then prepares to present her findings to the consultant.

'Mark is a 54-year-old tiler who presents with 2 days of upper abdominal pain with reduced oral intake. He has a history of peptic ulcer disease but is on no treatment. The pain worsened today and his wife drove him up here. He's exquisitely tender in his epigastric region with guarding and reduced bowel sounds. He's dehydrated, tachycardic and tachypnoeic and I've cannulated him and treated his pain with morphine. I've started a litre of normal saline. I'm concerned he has a perforated peptic ulcer and I've sent bloods for FBC, U&Es, LFTs, coagulation profile, and a group and hold. I'm organising an erect chest X-ray.'

The consultant agreed. 'That's a good plan. Make sure he's adequately resuscitated, and it might be worthwhile inserting a second IV line. He should have 80 mg of IV esomeprazole while we're waiting for the investigations.'

Clinical comment

The different causes of upper abdominal pain and the appropriate investigations can be summarised in Table 8.1 overleaf. Rather than taking a 'scattergun' approach to diagnosis and ordering every possible investigation, it is both clinically prudent and cost-effective to target investigations framed around the question 'How will this affect my diagnosis and management?' For example, a plain abdominal X-ray will not assist with the diagnosis in this instance—an erect chest X-ray, hepatobiliary ultrasound or computerised tomography (CT) scanning would be the most useful radiological investigations in this instance, depending upon the clinical suspicion.

Until a specific diagnosis is made, then, general supportive care should be provided. This includes providing adequate analgesia (which can facilitate examination rather than mask clinical signs), restoration of circulating blood volume with intravenous fluids, and keeping the patient fasted until a definitive plan is formulated. Absence of a diagnosis must not delay referral to the surgical or intensive care teams if a patient is shocked and critically ill.

Table 8.1 Selected causes of abdominal pain, characteristics, key investigations, and emergent management

Presenting features	Causes	Characteristics of diagnosis	Key investigations	Management
Upper abdominal pain	Perforated peptic ulcer	Tenderness, rigid guarded abdomen, shock	Erect chest X-ray looking for sub-diaphragmatic free gas	NG suction, triple antibiotics, urgent surgical referral
	Peptic ulcer disease	Little tenderness, response to therapy	Exclusion of other causes then upper GI endoscopy	Medical management with medication
	Pancreatitis	Tenderness, guarding, shock	Lipase, CT abdomen +/– hepatobiliary USS looking for signs of dilated biliary duct	Surgical referral +/– antibiotics, surgical debridement or ERCP if due to biliary calculus
Right upper quadrant pain, nausea and vomiting	Biliary colic	History, absence of inflammatory signs such as RUQ tenderness ('Murphy's sign') and fever	Liver function tests looking for signs of obstructive jaundice; then USS	Analgesia, dietary (avoid fats), elective cholecystectomy
RUQ pain, jaundice, rigors	Cholangitis	Fever and jaundice	FBC (elevated WCC), obstructive LFTs, USS showing dilated ducts	Antibiotic therapy, urgent ERCP

Mark's pain is returning just as he is being wheeled around to X-ray, so another 5 mg of intravenous morphine is administered. Allison writes up further fluid orders and goes to see another patient in the meantime. Realising that he will be admitted to hospital regardless of the diagnosis and that finding a bed can take some time, she submits a bed request to the administration staff.

11:35 hours

The chest X-ray has been completed (see Figure 8.1 below).

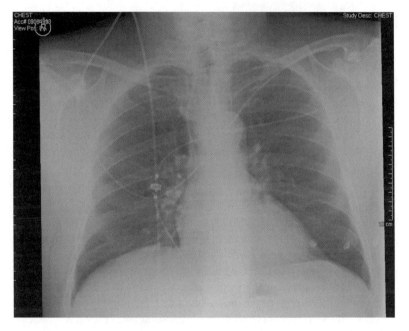

Figure 8.1: Erect chest X-ray

Allison and the consultant review the film together.

'Hmmm. No free gas under the diaphragm. I was expecting to see some. I guess that rules out a perforation.'

'No, it doesn't rule it out but it makes it less likely at this stage. If you're really concerned that he's perforated he should have a CT scan to confirm and you should start him on triple antibiotic therapy regardless.' The consultant paused. 'Is there anything else that could be causing his pain?'

Allison thought for a moment. 'He does drink 6 beers a day, and he does have some features of liver disease such as a few spider naevi and a palpable spleen. I wonder if he has some underlying cirrhosis and today's pain is due to pancreatitis?'

'Better ring the lab and ask them to add on a lipase and calcium then,' the consultant suggested.

Physiology comment

Pancreatitis can be defined as acute or chronic inflammation of the pancreas and can be caused by:

- Blockage of pancreatic ducts (gallstones, or protein plug formation) with secondary activation of digestive enzymes within the pancreatic acinar cells
- Toxic damage to the pancreas (alcohol) leading to autodigestion of organ reflux of bile or duodenal contents into the pancreatic ducts.

High levels of alcohol are toxic to the organ and may directly cause damage to the pancreas or may contribute to the development of pancreatitis by promoting protein deposition in the pancreatic ducts, thereby increasing the likelihood of blockage and recurrent inflammation. Blockage may also be caused by gallstones obstructing the movement of pancreatic juice into the small intestine. Blockage of the ducts by whatever mechanism leads to inappropriate activation of digestive enzymes, resulting in damage to the organ, often with far-ranging consequences. As in Mark's case, pancreatitis usually causes severe epigastric pain. The pain is often associated with vomiting as a consequence of irritation of the overlying stomach.

12:15 hours

The blood results have returned and are displayed on the screen in the department (see Table 8.2 opposite).

Table 8.2 Blood results

Result	Level	Normal range
Biochemistry		
Na	138	135–145 mmol/L
K	4.8	3.5–4.5 mmol/L
Cl	105	95–110 mmol/L
HCO$_3$	14	22–32 mmol/L
Urea	8.3	3.0–8.0 mmol/L
Creatinine	0.128	< 0.120 mmol/L
Anion gap	31	10–14 mmol/L
GGT	647	< 50 U/L
AST	1034	< 40 U/L
Lipase	2432	< 70 mmol/L
Ca (corr)	1.89	2.15–2.6 mmol/L
Haematology		
Hb	154	115–165 g/L
WCC	18.4	4.0–11.0 × 10^9/L
Neutrophils	15.3	–
Platelets	368	150–400 × 10^9/L

Physiology comment

Self-digestion of the pancreas initiates a large shift of protein and fluid from the plasma volume into the vascular space. This shift can be caused by the digestion of blood vessels within the gland leading to haemorrhage, and/or a widespread inflammatory response. Release of trypsin activates the complement and kinin cascades, leading to widespread clotting and shock. Phospholipase A2 may break down surfactant in the lung, leading to alveolar collapse and respiratory failure. The loss of fluid from the vascular space can lead to poor perfusion of the kidneys, with a result-ant rise in the indicators of renal function (urea and creatinine). Serum levels of the pancreatic enzymes are elevated as a result of leakage into the circulatory system from the inflamed pancreas.

Having seen the low bicarbonate on the blood results, Allison proceeds to take an arterial blood gas on room air (see Table 8.3 overleaf).

Table 8.3 Arterial blood gas results

Result	Level	Normal range
pH	7.31	7.35–7.45
pCO_2	17	35–45 mmHg
pO_2	74	80–100 mmHg
HCO_3	17	22–32 mmol/L
Base excess	–7.8	–3 – +3
Blood glucose	2.8	–
Lactate	5.3	<1.6

Physiology comment

The term 'anion gap' is a concept that is valuable in clinical acid–base evaluation. It provides an estimate of the difference between the commonly measured anions and cations in the blood.

The simplest of reports may only give the following, but they are still useful:

$$[Na^+] + [\text{other cations}] = [Cl^-] + [HCO_3^-] + [\text{other anions}]$$

$$[Na^+] - ([Cl^-] + [HCO3^-]) = [\text{other anions}] - [\text{other cations}]$$

$$= \text{anion gap}$$

When these values are compared in normal plasma, an apparent discrepancy of around 15 mmol/L is present (normal range = 8–16 mmol/L). This 'anion' gap is largely explained by the multiple negative charges found on some of the larger molecules (plasma proteins) present in the plasma. Evaluating the anion gap gives a simple tool to evaluate the cause of a metabolic acidosis. Where a mineral acid, such as HCl, accumulates in the body, or bicarbonate is lost, the drop in the bicarbonate is offset by a rise in the chloride (derived from the mineral acid) value. The net effect is that the anion gap remains unchanged. If, however, an organic acid such as a keto acid or lactate accumulates in the body, the bicarbonate will fall, but this fall will not be balanced by a rise in chloride. As the organic acid is not measured it adds to the anion gap, and the plasma chloride does not change from normal. Causes of increased anion gap and normal-pattern metabolic acidosis are given in Table 8.4 opposite.

Table 8.4 Causes of normal anion gap and increased anion gap metabolic acidosis

Causes of normal anion gap acidosis	Causes of increased anion gap metabolic acidosis
Ingestion of HCl or NH_4Cl	Diabetic ketoacidosis
Severe and or prolonged diarrhoea (loss of bicarbonate)	Starvation ketosis
	Lactic acidosis
Renal loss of bicarbonate	Methanol poisoning (formate)
Impaired renal acid secretion	Salicylate poisoning (salicylate)

In the case of Mark, who is suffering from pancreatitis, the metabolic acidosis with increased anion gap probably arises from one or both of the following mechanisms:

- Impaired renal function because the reduced circulating volume causes retention of organic acids
- Lactic acidosis due to the reduced circulating volume and consequent tissue hypoxia.

Clinical question 4

Interpret the results. Does this rule in or rule out any diagnosis?

Clinical comment

The markedly elevated lipase confirms a diagnosis of pancreatitis. However, the cause must be considered: most causes of acute pancreatitis in the Western world are attributable to alcohol and gallstones. The abnormal liver function tests could be caused by chronic alcohol abuse with liver dysfunction, or Mark could have a gallstone impacted in his common bile duct, producing biliary obstruction and the pancreatitis. The blood tests here show a significant inflammatory response with a raised white cell count, and the elevated anion gap and an acidaemia on the arterial blood gas suggest a metabolic acidosis. The low calcium suggests calcium sequestration as a result of saponification from liberated pancreatic enzymes. These bloods confirm that Mark is suffering from acute pancreatitis, and he is compromised as a result. A number of scoring systems such as Ranson's, APACHE II, and SOFA can grade the severity and assist with determining the prognosis of the condition. It is not sufficient to simply make the diagnosis—early identification of at-risk patients and referral to the intensive care unit is equally important. Complications could be expected in Mark's case because a number of poor prognostic features are present, such as an elevated WCC, hypocalcaemia, renal impairment, a metabolic acidosis, and clinical features of hypoperfusion. A CT scan should be performed to assist with risk stratification and to rule out co-existing pathologies.

An elevated anion gap occurs when there is a build-up of organic, inorganic, or exogenous acids. Causes of an elevated anion gap in the clinical setting can be remembered by the mnemonic MUDPILES:

- Methanol
- Uraemia
- Diabetic, alcoholic, and starvation ketoacidosis
- Paraldehyde
- Isoniazid and iron
- Lactic acidosis (pancreatitis is an important cause)
- Ethylene glycol
- Salicylates.

Hypocalcaemia can cause serious complications by itself: it can cause tetany (the involuntary contraction of muscles, due to increases in the action potential), laryngospasm, and cardiac arrhythmias. It is most commonly caused by hypoparathyroidism, vitamin D deficiency, and eating disorders.

Physiology comment

Calcium ions play a key role in many processes, including cell division, bone formation, blood coagulation, muscle contraction and neurotransmitter release. The total $[Ca^{2+}]$ in plasma is 2.5 mm/L, and its ECF concentration is normally very tightly regulated. In acute pancreatitis, hypocalcaemia may develop over time. The mechanism is multifactorial and is thought to include the removal of free calcium through the formation of calcium soaps. The calcium soaps are formed by the activity of activated lipase, often within the pancreas itself. Release of glucagon may also contribute to the lowered calcium levels. Glucagon stimulates the release of calcitonin, promoting bone uptake. It is thought that glucagon also will directly suppress the release of calcium from bone matrix (resorption). Hypocalcaemia increases the excitability of nerve and muscle cells, and leads to skeletal muscle spasms.

Allison administers one ampoule of 10% calcium gluconate intravenously, and then refers Mark to the surgical registrar while the consultant liaises with the intensive care unit (ICU). Mark is admitted to ICU once he has had a CT scan of his abdomen.

Physiology comment

Base excess can be defined as the amount of hydrogen ions required to return the pH of blood to 7.35 if the partial pressure of carbon dioxide is adjusted to normal. Comparison of the base excess with the reference range may assist in determining whether an acid–base disturbance has a respiratory, metabolic, or mixed metabolic–respiratory cause. Normal base excess values range between -2.3 and +2.3 mmol/L. A base excess value of more than +3 mmol/L indicates that a patient has blood that requires increased amounts of acid to return the pH to neutral, usually indicative of alkalosis, whereas a value below –3 usually indicates that the patient is acidotic, as excess acid needs to be removed from the blood to return the pH back to normal. As Mark is suffering from a metabolic acidosis we would expect his base excess to be lower than –3, which is the case.

Epilogue

Mark had a turbulent course in the intensive care unit, developing sepsis and multi-organ failure. He required a laparotomy to debride necrotic tissue and to drain an abscess that had formed. After 10 days of aggressive therapy he stabilised and was discharged to a ward bed, and then home 5 days later. He was followed up by the gastroenterology unit for his cirrhosis of the liver with portal hypertension, and with advice and assistance to cease drinking alcohol.

Tips

- Pancreatitis can lead to shock with multi-organ failure and should not be underestimated.
- Pancreatitis is diagnosed by biochemical tests, but the lipase can be within the normal range in some patients.
- Obstructive liver function tests in the presence of pancreatitis suggests that the diagnosis may be 'gallstone' pancreatitis, which is a surgical and gastroenterological emergency.
- A metabolic acidosis is not uncommon and represents shock.

References and further reading

1   American Gastroenterological Association. AGA Institute, Medical position statement on acute pancreatitis. *Gastroenterology* 2007; 132: 2019–21.
2   Casaletto, J.J. Differential diagnosis of metabolic acidosis. *Emerg Med Clin N Am* 2005; 23: 771–87.
3   Ranson, J.H.C. Diagnostic standards for acute pancreatitis. *World J Surg* 1997; 21: 136–42.
4   Vonlaufen, A., Wilson, J.S. & Apte, M.V. Molecular mechanisms of pancreatitis: Current opinion, *J Gastroenterol Hepatol* 2008; 23: 1339–48.
5   Whitcomb, D.C. Acute pancreatitis. *N Engl J Med* 2006; 354: 2142–50.

Case review

Basic science questions

1   Pancreatitis can be caused by which of the following?
   A   A high sodium diet
   B   Sitting still for long periods of time
   C   A high protein diet
   D   Cardiac hypertrophy
   E   Blockage of pancreatic ducts
2   Which statement regrading the anion gap is most correct?
   A   A normal plasma anion gap ranges from 1 to 5 mmol/L
   B   The anion gap would be increased in the case of HCl ingestion
   C   Salicylate poisoning would lead to an elevated anion gap
   D   Diarrhoea would lead to an increased anion gap
   E   A normal plasma anion gap ranges from 20 to 25 mmol/L
3   Which statement regarding base excess is most correct?
   A   A base excess value of more than +3 mmol/L is indicative of acidosis
   B   Base excess can be defined as the amount of bicarbonate needed to neutralise the plasma
   C   Base excess can be defined as the amount of bicarbonate present in plasma
   D   Base excess is unchanged when organic acids are added to plasma
   E   Base excess is calculated with the partial pressure of carbon dioxide adjusted to normal levels

Clinical questions

1   Match the following clinical features with the most likely diagnosis.
   A   Right upper quadrant pain with vomiting and nausea.
   B   Right upper quadrant pain with jaundice and fevers.

C Right upper quadrant pain with fever and a positive Murphy's sign.

D Epigastric pain with guarding and rebound.

E Epigastric pain with an elevated lipase and elevated bilirubin.

    (i) Cholecystitis

    (ii) Cholangitis

    (iii) Perforated peptic ulcer

    (iv) Gallstone pancreatitis

    (v) Biliary colic

2 Which of the following is not a recognised cause of pancreatitis?

A Alcohol consumption

B Gallstones

C Thiazide diuretics

D ACE inhibitors

E Pancreatic tumour causing obstruction

3 Which of the following is not a cause of a raised anion gap?

A Cardiac arrest

B Renal failure

C Diabetic ketoacidosis

D Diarrhoea

E Ethylene glycol ingestion

Case 9
Jane just couldn't breathe …

Jane had been an asthmatic since childhood and had always recovered well from her exacerbations, but this episode seemed worse than the others. She had started her action plan but today she wasn't responding to her usual treatment …

Clinical learning objectives

- Be able to recognise the clinical features of respiratory distress.
- Be able to classify the severity of an exacerbation of asthma.
- Describe emergency therapy based upon current guidelines for asthma management.
- Discuss the indications and precautions for initiating invasive ventilation.

Physiology learning objectives

- Describe the physiological abnormalities caused by asthma.
- Describe the appropriate use of spirometry during an acute asthma attack.
- Explain the physiological mechanism by which hypoxaemia and hypercapnia develop during an asthma attack.
- Describe the physiological mechanism by which a respiratory acidosis develops during an acute asthma attack.

Timeline

09:00	Recognising an impending exacerbation of her asthma, Jane follows her management plan and increases her preventer medication.
22:05	Jane cannot get her breath despite multiple uses of her reliever medication; calls ambulance.
22:17	Ambulance arrives, commences therapy.
22:28	Departs scene.
22:32	Becomes increasingly breathless and agitated en route to hospital; ambulance upgrades to category 1 and intensifies therapy; pre-notifies emergency department.
22:40	Arrives at hospital and is met by resuscitation team; assessment and management continues.
23:07	Little response to initial therapy, and Jane is getting increasingly tired and irritable; escalation in therapy.

09:00 hours

Jane could feel that her asthma was going to flare up: there was a lot of smoke in the air from the annual forestry burn-offs, and if she anticipated things getting worse she would always increase her inhaled corticosteroid therapy. She regularly monitors her asthma objectively with her peak flow meter: today the best she could do was 250 L per minute. Closing the windows to keep the smoke out and planning on staying indoors all day to minimise her exposure to the irritating smoke, she takes 50 mg of oral prednisolone in the expectation of her asthma getting worse throughout the day.

22:05 hours

It had been a tough day for Jane. The smoke had blown through, her throat was burning, and she was wheezing and coughing more and more. Her breathing difficulties had reduced in response to regular salbutamol administered via a spacer device, but by later in the day she was lasting only 2 hours before she needed more salbutamol. By 10 o'clock at night, having just taken a double dose of salbutamol and getting increasingly 'tight' and unable to speak more than a few words at a time, she asked her mother to ring an ambulance. She kept taking two puffs of her salbutamol puffer every five minutes until the ambulance arrived.

22:17 hours

The ambulance had been dispatched quickly in response to Jane's mother's call. The communications officer who took the call recognised this to be a severe attack and advised Jane to keep taking regular puffs of her medication.

Upon arrival, the paramedics assessed Jane to be distressed: she is tachypnoeic, can only talk in short phrases, and has a marked tracheal tug. She could barely speak, and she had widespread expiratory wheezes throughout her chest.

Clinical question 1

(a) Based upon the information so far, classify the severity of Jane's asthma.
(b) Describe the features of respiratory distress.
(c) Describe your initial management at this stage.

Clinical comment

Jane is clearly in respiratory distress: she does not have enough respiratory effort to speak properly, she is breathing fast, and in trying to breathe she is generating such significant negative intrathoracic pressures that her trachea is being physically pulled down further into her chest and the tissue between the intercostal spaces is being drawn in. All of these are features of respiratory distress. A classification of asthma severity provided in Table 9.1 takes these features into account.

Based upon this classification, it can be seen that Jane is suffering from a severe exacerbation of asthma, and intensive early management is indicated. This is particularly concerning because Jane has already implemented her action plan and her condition has deteriorated despite her early use of corticosteroid. The mainstay of therapy at this point is the use of constant nebulised salbutamol and intravenous salbutamol along with provision of adequate oxygenation. The use of multiple doses of nebulised anticholinergic therapy such as 500 µg ipratropium has been shown to be of benefit.

Table 9.1 Classification of asthma severity

Findings	Mild	Moderate	Severe and life-threatening
Talks in	Sentences	Phrases	Words
Pulse rate	< 100/min	100–120/min	> 120/min
Central cyanosis	Absent	May be present	Likely to be present
Wheeze intensity	Variable	Moderate to loud	Often quiet
PEF	> 75% predicted	50–75%	< 50%
FEV1	> 75% predicted	50–75%	< 50%
Oximetry on presentation			< 90%
Arterial blood gas	Not necessary	Not necessary	Necessary
Other investigations	Not required	May be required	Check for hypokalaemia CXR

Adapted from National Asthma Council 2006, Asthma Management Handbook, page 39

The paramedics recognise the seriousness of the situation and begin high flow oxygen via an oxygen mask immediately and start 5 mg of nebulised salbutamol. They obtain intravenous access and administer 250 µg of intravenous salbutamol and 200 mg of hydrocortisone. Jane is transferred onto the ambulance trolley and monitoring is applied. The initial observations are recorded:

- PR   140 bpm
- RR   40
- SpO_2 92% on 15 L/min via non-rebreather mask
- 'Alert but looking tired; audible wheezing'

22:28 hours

Jane is loaded into the ambulance for the trip to hospital. The paramedic rings through to the emergency department:

'We're en route with Jane, an 18-year-old student who has a severe attack of asthma. She's maintaining her oxygen saturations at 92% on high-flow oxygen, and she's having constant salbutamol nebulisers. She's also had 500 µg of IV salbutamol and 200 mg of IV hydrocortisone. We'll be there in 10 minutes.'

22:32 hours

En route to hospital Jane becomes more agitated and tries to remove the oxygen mask. Her wheeze is less audible. The paramedic ceases the salbutamol and inserts 5 mL of 1 : 1000 of adrenaline into the nebuliser. The driver turns on the lights and sirens and upgrades to a category 1 emergency.

Clinical question 2

As a doctor in the emergency department, describe how you would prepare for Jane's arrival. Consider which staff may be required. What might you be expecting to do?

Clinical comment

This is a medical emergency, and early notification from the ambulance allows the receiving emergency department time to prepare appropriate staff and to clear the resuscitation cubicles. Medication, infusions and equipment can be prepared prior to the patient's arrival (see Figure 9.1 overleaf). Additional staff, such as radiographers, anaesthetists and intensive care, can be forewarned. The respiratory physician on call could be notified and may attend. Roles such as team leader, airway doctor and procedure doctor should be allocated in advance. The 'worst case' scenario of a respiratory arrest should be anticipated: the airway doctor can mentally prepare by revising difficult airway drills, and the drugs and equipment for a rapid sequence induction can be prepared. The airway doctor needs to assemble and check equipment, and would also be revising the particular risks associated with initiating ventilation in an asthmatic: the high intrathoracic pressures lead to air trapping and a high risk of barotrauma if the patient is ventilated with too fast a rate or too high a tidal volume. At the same time, ventilation needs to be initiated quickly and efficiently due to the lack of any respiratory reserve and the associated risk of dangerous hypoxia. It can be very difficult to maintain the airway and provide ventilation by bag and mask technique because in practice extremely high airway pressures are required to ventilate such patients—maintaining an adequate seal between the mask and the patient's face can hence be difficult. Therefore the most experienced person available should be nominated to be the airway doctor.

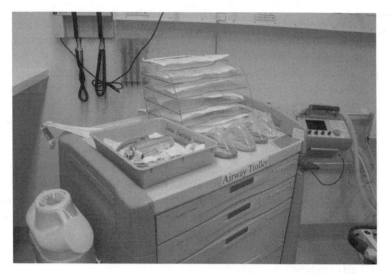

Figure 9.1 The pre-prepared airway trolley showing intubating equipment, masks and endotracheal tubes ready for use

Jane had difficulty talking in complete sentences, indicating severely reduced ventilatory capacity. This is an important indicator that if the attack continues to worsen it could become life-threatening. For this reason, her saturated oxygen level was monitored continuously with a pulse oximeter. As Jane was hypoxaemic, oxygen was administered simultaneously with nebulised bronchodilators.

Physiology comment

During an asthmatic attack the main physiological abnormality is high airway resistance, leading to reduced expiratory and inspiratory flows. This occurs through a combination of smooth muscle contraction (bronchoconstriction), inflammation of the airway wall, and mucus plugging. The increased resistance to breathing can lead to hyperinflation, and as a consequence to an abnormally large total lung capacity (TLC). An important feature of asthma that helps to distinguish it from other diseases that cause airway obstruction, notably chronic obstructive pulmonary disease (COPD), is that it is usually intermittent, and lung function often returns to normal or near normal between attacks. However, patients who have recurrent attacks (i.e. chronic asthmatics) can develop persistent airway obstruction with incomplete reversibility to bronchodilator therapy.

The common features of airway obstruction seen in asthma are reductions in FEV_1, FEV_1/FVC ratio, PEF, and a concavity in the descending limb of the expiratory flow–volume curve. In more severe cases the FVC is also reduced because the already narrowed airways close prematurely during the expiration, trapping gas in the lungs and resulting in a raised residual volume (RV). In the emergency setting it is not always easy to obtain spirometry in distressed patients with significant airway obstruction, but if it can be obtained the results help to assess the severity of the attack and subsequently the effectiveness of therapy. Under these conditions it is often easier to obtain a measurement of PEF, as this test only requires the patient to blow maximally (from TLC) for a couple of seconds. Peak expiratory flow can then be used to grade severity, particularly in children and young adults where other causes of airway obstruction such as COPD are unlikely, and to monitor progression and response to therapy.

22:40 hours

Jane arrives in the emergency department. The nebulised adrenaline has just finished and she has improved: she is more alert and can talk in short phrases again. She is transferred across to the trolley and the paramedics provide handover. Monitoring is applied, and her assessment and management starts. A nebuliser mask is applied and the salbutamol is continued. Jane is too breathless to speak any more than a few words at a time, so her mother provides a brief history.

'Jane's been an asthmatic since she was 3 and it's usually been well controlled with a regular preventer and a reliever when she needs it. It usually flares up when there's a lot of smoke in the air like today. She was hospitalised once, but exacerbations usually settle with a short course of prednisolone. She took 50 mg of prednisolone this morning and she tried to avoid the smoke today but she wouldn't settle. It worsened tonight and here we are.'

The vital signs are recorded and a directed examination is performed:

- PR   150 bpm
- RR   50
- BP   100/40
- Temp   36.5°C
- SpO_2 91% on oxygen
- Looks exhausted
- Talking in words only, intercostal recession

- Trachea midline
- Quiet chest, scattered wheezes throughout both lung fields; and no crackles.

A second intravenous line is inserted and blood tests collected; an arterial blood gas is taken (see Figure 9.2 below).

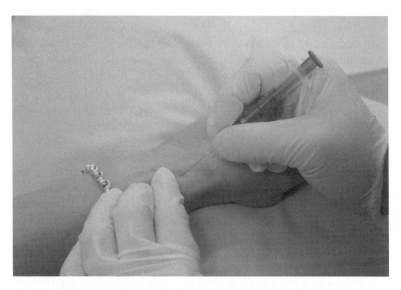

Figure 9.2 A small gauge needle is used to collect blood from the radial artery

Clinical question 3

(a) Summarise the findings so far. What additional therapy would you commence?

(b) What findings would you expect on the arterial blood gas?

Clinical comment

As expected from the information provided by the ambulance crew, Jane has a severe exacerbation of asthma. Aggressive therapy is required immediately—indeed, the paramedics administered nebulised adrenaline, which appears to have improved the situation in the short term. Part of the team's preparation is likely to have involved drawing up more nebulised salbutamol and adrenaline, and preparing an intravenous salbutamol infusion. In addition, a trial of non-invasive ventilation may improve the respiratory function of some asthmatics, so having such equipment on standby is warranted.

At this point continuing with the intravenous salbutamol via a continuous infusion is recommended. Bronchodilation may be improved by adding 500 µg of ipratropium to the salbutamol. The addition of nebulised magnesium as a bronchodilator in severe asthma has been proved, and should be used in this instance. The inspired oxygen should be maximised, but this can be difficult to maintain when nebulised medication is being administered, because the nebuliser requires only 6–8 L per minute of oxygen flow. Hypoxia may occur because oxygen delivery is inadequate when the nebuliser is being used; so additional oxygen should be provided by an additional catheter.

The arterial blood gas is performed to assess both oxygen exchange and ventilator function. Given that Jane can only manage oxygen saturations at 91–92% on high-flow oxygen, a large $p_{(A-a)}O_2$ gradient would be expected. Also, an acute respiratory acidosis would be expected to be seen because the poor ventilation results in a high pCO_2.

Jane has been receiving constant nebulised salbutamol since the ambulance arrived at her house. She is receiving an infusion of intravenous salbutamol, and a dose of nebulised magnesium made little difference. A mobile chest X-ray showed hyperinflated lung fields but no consolidation or pneumothorax.

The arterial blood gas result is displayed in Table 9.2 below.

Table 9.2 Arterial blood gas result

Result	Level	Normal range
FIO$_2$: 0.8 (estimated)		
pH	7.13	7.35–7.45
pCO$_2$	72	35–45 mmHg
pO$_2$	74	80–100 mmHg
HCO$_3$	18	22–32 mmol/L
Base excess	−5.8	−3–+3
K	3.6	3.5–4.5 mmol/L

Clinical comment

As expected, the blood gas reveals an acute respiratory acidosis. There appears to be an element of metabolic acidosis present as well (as evidenced by the low bicarbonate and a base deficit of –5.8). This is most likely due to a lactic acidosis produced by a degree of poor peripheral perfusion resulting from the systemic illness. Significantly, the pO_2 is low at 74 mmHg despite the high inspired oxygen concentration—even though by referring to the oxygen–haemoglobin dissociation curve this would provide an oxygen saturation reading above 90%, this is most concerning as there is very little reserve. Assuming the FIO_2 is 0.8, applying the alveolar gas equation gives a very elevated alveolar–arterial oxygen gradient of over 380 mmHg. Do not be reassured by the SpO_2 'in the 90s'—should Jane deteriorate further, the next step would be to intubate and ventilate with 100% oxygen. In fact, the staff should be anticipating the imminent need for invasive ventilation and be preparing for a rapid sequence induction.

It is important to note that Jane's potassium is relatively low considering the circumstances, and that there are competing processes occurring: the acidosis would move potassium out of the cells into the extracellular space, yet the constant salbutamol and the use of corticosteroids would be trying to move potassium the other way into the intracellular space (recall that salbutamol is the first line treatment for hyperkalaemia). Close monitoring and potassium replacement will be necessary.

Physiological comment

During an asthma attack, increased airway resistance results in reduced expiratory and to some extent inspiratory flows of all lung volumes. Hyperinflation can occur because narrowed small airways close prematurely or take too long to 'empty' during tidal breathing, a problem that is compounded by a high respiratory rate. Hyperinflation can have a positive effect on airway calibre as it imposes greater traction forces on the small airways, and this helps to hold them open. However, this is to some extent offset by the increased work of breathing, which may result in respiratory muscle fatigue and distress.

Indicators of a severe attack requiring urgent treatment include:

- Inability to speak in complete sentences
- Cyanosis

- Tachycardia
- Pulsus paradoxicus.

During an asthma attack, the degree of airway narrowing or closure is not uniform across all airways, and some gas exchange regions of the lung receive little, if any, ventilation. Although some compensatory redistribution of blood flow away from the poorly ventilated regions does occur, this maybe inadequate, with these units still receiving significant blood flow relative to ventilation so that unequal ventilation and perfusion results. This causes a widening of the alveolar–arterial oxygen gradient and reduced arterial oxygenation (hypoxaemia). A further decrease in arterial oxygenation may be seen following the administration of bronchodilators despite a reduction in airway resistance, an effect that is usually attributed to further increases in blood flow to poorly ventilated units. The p_aCO_2 commonly decreases during a mild attack or in the early phase of an attack in consequence of the overall high alveolar ventilation (hyperventilation) in response to hypoxic stimulation of ventilation as well as anxiety. However, an abnormally high p_aCO_2 (and fall in pH) can develop if the severity of the asthma attack worsens, and this is a clear indication of life-threatening asthma. The rising p_aCO_2 is due to respiratory muscle fatigue and incipient respiratory failure.

23:07 hours

Despite the aggressive therapy detailed earlier, Jane is looking worse. She is unable to speak at all, she is tired, and she is becoming drowsy (see Figure 9.3 overleaf). A repeat blood gas is taken as the staff prepare to intubate and ventilate (see Table 9.3 below).

Table 9.3 Repeat blood gas results

Result	Level	Normal range
FIO$_2$: 0.8 (estimated)		
pH	7.05	7.35–7.45
pCO$_2$	104	35–45 mmHg
pO$_2$	63	80–100 mmHg
HCO$_3$	16	22–32 mmol/L
Base excess	–6.1	–3 – + 3

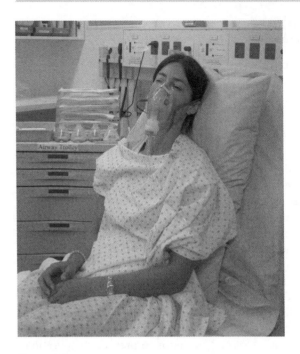

Figure 9.3

Physiology comment

The respiratory acidosis seen in severe cases of asthma is caused by the p_aCO_2 increasing as a result of respiratory muscle fatigue and incipient respiratory failure. The $HCO_3 : p_aCO_2$ ratio is reduced, and this depresses the pH. If respiratory acidosis persists, the kidney will respond by conserving bicarbonate. The resulting increase in plasma bicarbonate will then move the $HCO_3 : p_aCO_2$ ratio back towards its normal level. In Jane's case it is clear that the attack is severe as the pH has dropped significantly, indicating marked hypoventilation. Because the attack is acute, the renal system has not had time to respond by reabsorbing additional bicarbonate, so the respiratory acidosis can be classified as uncompensated. A base excess value below −3 (see Case 8) usually indicates that the patient is acidotic, as excess acid needs to be removed from the blood to return the pH back to normal. As Jane is suffering from an uncompensated respiratory acidosis we would expect her base excess to be lower than −3, which is the case.

Clinical question 4

(a) What would you do now?
(b) Interpret the second blood gas.

Clinical comment

Jane is displaying the clinical features of life-threatening asthma. It could be argued that the second blood gas was unnecessary as it would not change clinical management. She is tiring, and the blood gas shows worsening oxygenation and ventilation. She is on the verge of a respiratory arrest, and intubation should be performed without delay. It is essential that once intubation occurs she is ventilated by hand and at a slow rate—if she is placed on to a standard fixed-rate and fixed-volume transport ventilator there is a risk that she will develop barotrauma. More advanced ventilators with pressure control mechanisms will be required, and these are usually only used in the intensive care unit. The main aim of initiating invasive ventilation in this instance is to provide adequate oxygenation. A secondary aim is to prevent complications. Hence, permitting hypercapnoea for as long as it takes to overcome the profound bronchospasm should be a principle of management. This could take days of careful intensive care management.

Epilogue

Jane was intubated and was transferred to the intensive care unit. She received ongoing intensive therapy, but it still took 48 hours for her CO_2 to return to normal and for her ventilatory pressures to normalise. Once her oxygen requirements had decreased she was extubated and transferred to a ward, and was discharged home 3 days later. She was advised to be wary of specific triggers and to seek medical advice as soon as her symptoms worsened.

Tips

- Early recognition of life-threatening asthma and treating aggressively and appropriately can reduce mortality.
- Prepare for intubation and assemble senior staff in anticipation.

- The constant use of bronchodilators is essential.
- Do not rely solely on blood gases for assessment; use clinical criteria and frequent reassessment of the clinical state to guide management.

References and further reading

1   British Thoracic Society. Scottish Intercollegiate Guidelines Network. 6 Management of acute asthma. *Thorax* 2008; 63 (IV Supp): iv51–iv60.
2   Johns, D.P. & Pierce, R. *Pocket guide to spirometry*, 2nd edn, McGraw-Hill Australia, Sydney, 2007.
3   National Asthma Council. *Asthma management handbook*. South Melbourne, 2006. (Available at www.nationalasthma.org.au)
4   Rodrigo, G.J. & Castro-Rodriguez, J.A. Anticholinergics in the treatment of children and adults with acute asthma: A systematic review with meta-analysis. *Thorax* 2005; 60: 740–6. doi: 10.1136/thx.2005.047803
5   Rowe, B. & Camargo, C. Emergency department treatment of severe acute asthma. *Ann Emerg Med* 2006; 47: 564–66.
6   Rowe, B.H. & Wedzicha, J.A. Non-invasive positive pressure ventilation for treatment of respiratory failure due to severe acute exacerbations of asthma, Cochrane Database of Systematic Reviews 2005; Issue 3. Art. No.: CD004360. doi: 10.1002/14651858.CD004360.pub3
7   Silverman, R.A., Osborn, H., Runge, J., Gallagher, E.J. et al. IV magnesium sulfate in the treatment of acute severe asthma: A multicenter randomized controlled trial. Chest 2002; 122: 489–97.

Case review

Basic science questions

1   In asthma the main physiological abnormality is:
   A   Reduced airway resistance
   B   Increased chest wall compliance
   C   Reduced chest wall compliance
   D   Increased airway resistance
   E   Alveolar destruction

2   The common features of spirometry in asthma are:
   A   Reductions in FEV_1, FEV_1/FVC ratio and PEF
   B   Reductions in FEV_1, FEV_1/FVC ratio and an increase in PEF
   C   Increases in FEV_1, FEV_1/FVC ratio and PEF
   D   Increases in FEV_1, FEV_1/FVC ratio and a reduction in PEF
   E   Unchanged spirometry

3 An additional decrease in arterial oxygenation may be seen following the administration of bronchodilators in asthma due to which of the following?

A Reflex bronchoconstriction
B A lowering of the ventilation rate
C Fatigue of the accessory muscles of ventilation
D Reflex tachycardia
E Further increases in blood flow to poorly ventilated units

Clinical questions

1 Classify the following asthma exacerbations according to their severity.

A Breathless, occasional wheeze, talking in sentences, and PEF > 75% predicted.
B Semi-conscious, tachycardic and cyanosed.
C Breathless, talking in words, and a quiet chest with no wheeze.
D Breathless, talking in phrases, widespread wheeze, and PEF > 50% predicted.
  (i) Mild
  (ii) Moderate
  (iii) Severe
  (iv) Life-threatening

2 Which of the following therapies are not indicated in severe asthma exacerbations?

A Intravenous magnesium
B Intravenous salbutamol
C Leukotriene receptor antagonists
D Non-invasive ventilation
E Nebulised adrenaline

Case 10
No one knows who he is and why he's so unwell ...

Medical and nursing staff are called to the resuscitation bay late at night as paramedics bring this patient into the department. No one knows his name, or the circumstances surrounding his presentation. Whatever the case, you have to commence resuscitation and rapidly make the diagnosis. Your accumulated knowledge of metabolic matters will aid greatly ...

Clinical learning objectives

- Describe how to assess an unconscious patient.
- Describe the emergency management of an unconscious patient.
- Understand the common causes of a reduced level of consciousness.
- Be able to utilise pathology tests to diagnose the cause of a reduced level of consciousness and stratify risk.

Physiology learning objectives

- Define the term 'mixed acid–base disorder' and understand how a metabolic acidosis and respiratory alkalosis can arise from certain conditions.
- Describe how acidosis alters internal potassium balance.
- Describe how to calculate a plasma anion gap and why certain conditions lead to an increased anion gap.
- Understand how alkalinisation of the urine increases the urinary excretion of selected drugs.

Timeline

23:32	Paramedics arrive as a category 1; handover occurs and resuscitation begins.
23:45	Patient's airway secured, arterial blood gas and bloods taken and sent to pathology.
23:52	Arterial blood gas results available, 12-lead ECG obtained, supportive care continues.
00:34	Patient transferred to CT scanner.
00:57	Initial blood and radiological results available.
01:35	Further results available; specific treatment starts.
03:27	Patient transferred to the intensive care unit for continuing treatment.

23:32 hours

It's late at night and you've seen a lot of patients today. It shouldn't be long before you can hand over to the night team and go home for a well-earned rest. Just as you're in the process of discharging your last patient, the triage nurse's voice comes through loudly on the public address system: 'resuscitation staff to resus; resuscitation staff to resus'. You and the registrar rush to the resuscitation bay to find the paramedics moving a motionless male patient on to the bed. He is barely breathing, and requires assistance to maintain his airway and breathing. The paramedic provides the handover:

> 'We were called to a house as a collapse … we found him lying on the floor, barely breathing and with a pulse rate of 130, a blood pressure of 80/50 and a GCS of 6 … we've cannulated him and commenced IV fluids, and we're supporting his As and Bs with the bag and mask. He's tolerated a Gueddel's, and there's been an improvement in his blood pressure after 500 millilitres of Hartmann's.'

The paramedics depart as the medical team takes over and continues management. Monitoring is applied and the individual team members take their positions around the patient.

The initial signs are recorded:

- PR   130 bpm
- BP   100 / 60
- RR   26 and shallow; airway not maintained spontaneously

- SpO$_2$ 95% on oxygen
- GCS 5—E1   V2 M2 Pupils equal, 3 mm diameter
- Temp   37.4°C
- Patient cool, poorly perfused with dry lips and tongue
- Smells of alcohol

Clinical question 1

(a) What are the issues to consider in the initial assessment and management of this patient?

(b) Describe your initial actions and list your differential diagnoses.

Clinical comment

The initial assessment and management of an unconscious patient is directed towards resuscitation—that is, the patient must be kept alive while the cause of the condition is sought. The absence of an immediate diagnosis must not delay the commencement of life-saving resuscitation treatment. The primary survey identifies immediate threats to life, and as applied to this patient:

- The patient is not maintaining an adequate airway and requires manual support. The ability to maintain an airway using simple means such as a bag and mask device and an oropharyngeal airway is essential and life-saving, and can be administered by anyone. The patient may require tracheal intubation to secure the airway definitively, but this should only be performed by personnel experienced in such procedures. Non-invasive techniques will keep patients alive until a definitive procedure can be performed safely.
- His breathing is rapid and shallow and may not be sufficient to maintain adequate oxygenation and ventilation, hence he may require assisted breaths with a bag and mask device.
- His circulation is compromised as evidenced by cool peripheries, tachycardia, and a low blood pressure. His condition improved with the prehospital administration of 500 mL of intravenous crystalloid fluid. This should continue into the emergency department.

Medical staff should be considering the possible causes of the reduced level of consciousness when assessing such patients. The smell of alcohol on the patient's breath was noted by the treating team, but it should never be assumed that this is the primary and only cause for a reduced level of consciousness. There are a wide variety of possible diagnoses, each with markedly different clinical features and treatments. The mnemonic 'AEIOU TIPS' provides a ready means to recall the possible causes:

A Alcohol and other toxins
E Endocrinopathy
   Encephalopathy
   Electrolyte disturbances
I Insulin—diabetes
O Oxygen—hypoxia of any cause
   Opiates
U Uraemia
T Trauma
I Infection
P Psychogenic
S Seizure
   Syncope
   Space-occupying lesion

With the principles of resuscitation and a brief overview of possible causes in your mind, you proceed with your assessment and management.

The patient looks unwell, and his mental state has not improved following the administration of intravenous fluid. A brief and necessarily limited neurological examination does not reveal any localising deficits—his reflexes are equal, and he has normal tone on both left and right sides. There is no rash to suggest meningococcaemia. A further 1 L of 0.9% NaCl is commenced via the intravenous cannula placed by the paramedic. The registrar has taken up position at the patient's head and is administering 100% oxygen via a tight-fitting oxygen mask with a bag and valve, and directs you to insert another cannula in the patient's right antecubital fossa. You easily obtain access and withdraw 20 millilitres of blood from the cannula and place it into pathology tubes. You also take an arterial blood gas from the patient's left radial artery.

Clinical question 2

(a) What blood tests would you request? Justify your choices.
(b) What would you expect to see on the ABG?
(c) What should happen now?

23:45 hours

Despite basic supportive care being provided, the patient has not improved and remains critically ill. He is not supporting his airway and his breathing appears to be inadequate. The decision to definitively secure the patient's airway is made, and the registrar proceeds to perform a rapid sequence intubation using sedation with 100 µg of fentanyl and 2 mg of midazolam and muscle relaxation with 100 mg of suxamethonium. A size 7.5 endo–tracheal tube passes easily into the trachea, and it is tied at the patient's lips at the 22 cm mark. The patient is placed onto a ventilator with a respiratory rate of 12 and a tidal volume of 800 mL, and continuing muscle relaxation is provided with 50 mg rocuronium boluses and an infusion of morphine and midazolam.

Now that the airway is secured, a more detailed examination commences. There is no rash, and the chest is clear with equal air entry. There are no features consistent with the presence of chronic liver disease. No obvious toxidromes are present, in that there are no clinical features of anticholinergic or cholinergic poisoning apparent. There are no palpable masses in the abdomen, and no external signs of trauma to the head or trunk.

The blood tubes are sent to the pathology laboratory with the following requests:

- FBC
- U&Es
- LFTs
- Blood cultures
- Serum paracetamol and ethanol levels.

23:52 hours

A 12-lead ECG is performed and the results from the ABG taken pre-intubation become available (see Table 10.1 and Figure 10.1 overleaf). The intravenous fluid continues and there has been little change in the clinical situation.

Table 10.1 Arterial blood gas results

Result	Level	Normal range
FIO$_2$: 1.00		
pH	7.29	7.35–7.45
pCO$_2$	12	35–45 mmHg
pO$_2$	453	80–100 mmHg
HCO$_3$	17	22–32 mmol/L
Base excess	−11.8	−3 – +3
Blood glucose	3.8	–
Lactate	8.3	<1.6

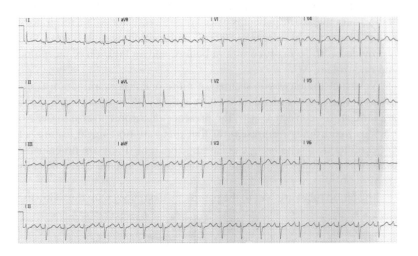

Figure 10.1 12-lead ECG

Clinical question 3

Interpret the ECG and the ABG. Have these provided any clues to the diagnosis?

Physiology comment

As discussed in Case 2, a metabolic acidosis is characterised by an initial drop in plasma pH that is blunted by the body's physicochemical buffer systems, leading to a decrease in plasma $[HCO_3]$. Over a matter of hours, as long as it is able, the rate and depth of ventilation will increase, leading to a drop in the $[pCO_2]$ to compensate. Over the longer term, the plasma $[HCO_3]$ will begin to rise back towards normal as the kidneys excrete $[H^+]$ and in so doing add $[HCO_3]$ to the plasma.
Case values:

- pH   7.23
- pCO_2 12
- HCO_3 12

The case values indicate that an acidaemia is indeed present: both the plasma $[HCO_3]$ and $[pCO_2]$ values are depressed, indicating a metabolic acidosis. Of note is the $[pCO_2]$, which is lower than would be expected as a result of respiratory compensation alone. This suggests that another acid–base disorder is superimposed upon the underlying metabolic acidosis, leading to a mixed disorder. Together with clinical information, the pH, plasma $[HCO_3]$ and $[pCO_2]$ are sufficient to diagnose uncomplicated single acid–base disturbances. In fact a series of rules can be used to predict compensatory changes in $[HCO_3]$ and $[pCO_2]$ for each uncomplicated acid–base disorder (see clinical comment). When the ABG data is not consistent with these rules, a mixed acid–base disorder can be inferred (see below).

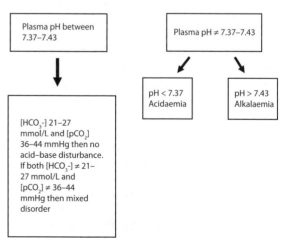

Mixed acid–base disorders are those in which two or more primary aetiological disorders are present simultaneously. In acetylsalicylic acid poisoning, significant hyperventilation often occurs as a result of direct stimulation of the respiratory centre. Indirect stimulation of ventilation can also be caused by an increased production of CO_2 as a result of salicylate-induced uncoupling of oxidative phosphorylation. Respiratory alkalosis therefore develops alongside the metabolic acidosis induced by acetylsalicylic acid, leading to 2 aetiological disorders causing the acid–base disturbance; hence the classification of a mixed disorder. Renal compensation will lead to bicarbonate excretion, often accompanied by sodium, potassium and water loss. Loss of bicarbonate reduces the body's buffering capacity, allowing the further development of the metabolic acidosis.

Clinical comment

The lack of a history from the patient or a collateral history denies treating clinicians a traditional starting point, and therefore physical and laboratory examination becomes critical. However, the physical examination has not provided any immediate clues, such as an obvious sign of a head injury, that could explain such a clinical presentation. It is important to note that such an injury is not ruled out by this, and that an urgent CT scan of the brain will be required to assess for an intracerebral event.

Some blood tests will play an important role in the assessment of this patient. Nevertheless, as with all pathology requests, treating doctors must be able to justify reasons for all tests rather than conducting a broad sweep in the hope of identifying any pathology. In this instance, the biochemistry tests can be justified by wishing to assess for toxicological causes and electrolyte abnormalities. Abnormal liver function tests would alert the treating team to the possibility of liver failure and hepatic encephalopathy, and a full blood count may reveal signs of inflammation, which may suggest underlying infection as a cause.

The ABG can play a key role in assessing this patient by diagnosing acid–base abnormalities. With low bicarbonate, a large base deficit and an elevated lactate level, there is obviously a profound metabolic acidosis present. However, this ABG result is surprising in that the pCO_2 is lower than you would expect if it were purely a result of respiratory compensation to the metabolic acidosis. This consequently makes the pH higher than you would expect if the profound metabolic acidosis alone were present. This subtle result raises the possibility that there is another process present producing a primary respiratory alkalosis. An overview of acid–base disorders and some rule-of-thumb compensation calculations are provided in Table 10.2 below. Additionally, the blood glucose is relatively low at 3.8 mmol/L.

Table 10.2 Primary changes and compensations in simple acid–base disorders

Disorder	pH	HCO$_3$	pCO$_2$	Compensation
Metabolic acidosis	< 7.36	Primary decrease	Compensatory decrease	1.2 mmHg decrease in pCO$_2$ for every 1 mmol/L decrease in HCO$_3$
Metabolic alkalosis	> 7.44	Primary increase	Compensatory increase	0.6–0.75 mmHg increase in pCO$_2$ for every 1 mmol/L increase in HCO$_3$. pCO$_2$ should not rise above 60 mmHg in compensation
Respiratory acidosis	< 7.36	Compensatory increase	Primary increase	Acute: 1–2 mmol increase in HCO$_3$ for every 10 mmHg increase in pCO$_2$ Chronic: 3–4 mmol increase in HCO$_3$ for every 10 mmHg increase in pCO$_2$
Respiratory alkalosis	> 7.44	Compensatory decrease	Primary decrease	Acute: 1–2 mmol decrease in HCO$_3$ for every 10 mmHg decrease in pCO$_2$ Chronic: 4–5 mmol decrease in HCO$_3$ for every 10 mmHg decrease in pCO$_2$

The ECG can be useful in making a diagnosis—arrhythmias can be identified; changes consistent with anticholinergic poisoning must be looked for specifically, and, if present, these will alert the clinicians that this class of drugs may be involved as a cause. In this circumstance, there is nothing specific that suggests such a diagnosis. The tachycardia, while important to note, is non-specific by itself and can be explained by the patient's clinical state.

The treating team continues fluid resuscitation and increases the respiratory rate on the ventilator to compensate adequately for the metabolic acidosis shown on the ABG. An indwelling catheter is introduced into the bladder so that the urine output can be measured accurately in 'real time'. The registrar reviews progress so far:

'He's unconscious, smells of alcohol, but has a metabolic acidosis and possibly another process present. His blood sugar level is at the lower level of normal, so let's administer 25 mL of 50% dextrose. We can't rule out an intracranial event as a cause for this, and there may be another toxin present, such as salicylates … let's organise a CT brain and request salicylate levels … in the meantime, let's continue with the intravenous fluids and re-check his ABG … and regardless of the cause, we'd better notify the intensive care unit so that they can start organising a bed.'

00:34 hours

The registrar calls in his consultant to supervise the department while he is away in the radiology department, and the team prepares to escort the patient to the CT scanner. Prior to transfer, the registrar and the nursing staff check their equipment for the transfer—it is essential that any eventuality be anticipated and prepared for. They collect supplies of resuscitation and intubation drugs, and check basic and advanced airway equipment so they are prepared in case of an accidental extubation or deterioration in the patient's clinical state away from the emergency department.

The patient is escorted to the scanner by the emergency registrar and nurse, and an orderly. The transfer is uneventful and the patient returns to the department to continue treatment and await results.

00:57 hours

The initial blood results become available (see Table 10.3 opposite).

Table 10.3 Blood results

Result	Level	Normal range
Biochemistry		
Na	135	135–145 mmol/L
K	5.8	3.5–4.5 mmol/L
Cl	98	95–110 mmol/L
HCO_3	12	22–32 mmol/L
Urea	14.3	3.0–8.0 mmol/L
Creatinine	0.138	< 0.120 mmol/L
Anion gap	31	10–14 mmol/L
GGT	–	< 50 U/L
AST	–	< 40 U/L
Haematology		
Hb	154	130–180 g/L
WCC	4.7	$4.0–11.0 \times 10^9$/L
Platelets	210	$150–400 \times 10^9$/L
Special pathology		
Paracetamol	< 22 µmol/L	
Salicylate	Pending	
Ethanol	65 mmol/L	

The radiology registrar rings the emergency registrar to inform him that no abnormality is seen on the CT scan.

Clinical question 4

(a) Given these results, what are the most likely diagnoses?

(b) Describe how you will proceed with treatment.

Physiology comment

Internal potassium balance describes how the total body pool of potassium is distributed between the intracellular and extracellular compartments.

The concentration of potassium is typically high in cells (150 mmol/L) and low in the extracellular fluid (4.5 mmol/L), with the difference being governed primarily by the activity of membrane-bound energy-dependent NaK pumps and the relative permeability to potassium of the cell membrane itself. A range of factors, including insulin, circulating catecholamine levels, aldosterone and pH, can influence the internal balance of potassium and cause movement in to or out of cells.

Fluctuations in the extracellular $[H^+]$ have the potential to alter the internal balance of potassium, and therefore have a profound effect on the plasma potassium concentration. As a rule, an acidosis will lead to a rise in the plasma potassium concentration as hydrogen ions and potassium ions exchange for each other across the cell membrane. In reality, however, some acid–base disturbances cause little or no alteration in internal potassium balance, whereas others have much more of an effect. Respiratory acid–base disorders as well as metabolic acidoses that are caused by organic acids (such as lactate) do not cause major changes in the internal balance of potassium, whereas metabolic acidoses caused by mineral acids often elicit large shifts in potassium. This can be explained by the differing properties of the associated anions. If the anion such as chloride is unable to penetrate the cell membrane, then exchange with potassium will occur, because the entry of H^+ into the cell upsets the electrical neutrality, generating an electrical gradient that promotes potassium efflux. If the associated anion, such as lactate, does penetrate the cell membrane, then the intracellular electrical balance remains unaltered and little change in the internal balance of potassium occurs. In a respiratory acidoses, carbon dioxide is able to diffuse readily into the cell, forming carbonic acid and in turn H^+ and HCO_3^-, causing little movement of K^+ as little change in electrical neutrality occurs.

The registrar reviews the results and considers the possibilities.

'There's an elevated anion gap, along with a mixed acid–base picture and no other cause—it has to be salicylates. Activated charcoal may be of benefit in this case. Let's alkalinise the urine and await the level; we may need to consider dialysis …'

Physiology comment

As the plasma is electrically neutral, the number of negative equivalents (a measure of the number of available charges) always balances the equivalents of anions. By tradition, however, not every ionic constituent is reported in laboratory results, and so, when the plasma concentrations of the major cations (Na^+ and K^+) and the measured anions ($Cl-$ and HCO_3^-) are compared, a difference or 'gap' of approximately 15 mmol/L arises. This anion gap therefore gives a measure of the difference between the main reported anions and cations. Review of the anion gap is of particular use in the differential diagnosis of metabolic acidosis. An increased anion gap indicates the presence of excess unmeasured anions in solutions (usually conjugate bases of the acids that have entered the system). Thus:

$$([Na^+] + [K^+]) - ([Cl^-] + [HCO_3^-]) = [\text{other anions}] - [\text{other cations}]$$
$$= \text{anion gap}$$

Aspirin or acetylsalicylic acid has an acid dissociation constant (pKa) of 3.5 at 25°C, meaning that it will be only partially dissociated in biological systems. However, when acetylsalicylic acid is present in large enough amounts, it leads to an increased anion gap as the measured bicarbonate is replaced by the unmeasured conjugate base (salicylate) anions. Taking large amounts of aspirin uses up bicarbonate (taking $Na^+ = 140$, $K^+ = 4$, $HCO_3^- = 22$ and $Cl^- = 105$, for example), such that the HCO_3^- value can fall from approximately 22 to about 10 mmol/L, thereby raising the anion gap from approximately 17 to about 29 mmol/L.

The registrar writes up further drugs, fluids and sodium bicarbonate to achieve urinary alkalinisation (see Table 10.4 below).

Table 10.4 Drugs, fluids and bicarbonate

Fluid	Amount	Additives	Rate
5% dextrose	1000 mL	100 mL $NaHCO_3$	250 mL/h
N/S	1000 mL	–	125 mL/h
Activated charcoal	50 g	NG	–

Clinical comment

It is increasingly likely that a severe acid–base disorder is responsible for this patient's condition. This was evident in the ABG result, but additionally it can be seen that there is an elevated anion gap, as calculated by subtracting the chloride and bicarbonate results from the sodium and the potassium results. The anion gap is thus calculated to be 31.

The causes for such a disturbance in acid–base balance are varied, but very few conditions cause a mixed acid–base disorder. Intoxication with alcohol will produce these clinical findings and a metabolic acidosis, but this alone will not explain the mixed picture. Salicylate poisoning must be suspected, and in the presence of a normal CT brain and no other immediate cause for such an acidosis, treatment should be directed towards treating this serious overdose.

01:35 hours

The laboratory technician rings through with the eagerly awaited salicylate result: it is 6.7 mmol/L, with the normal range being between 1.1 and 2.2 mmol/L. The diagnosis is thus confirmed, and now the management can be specifically directed towards treating this dangerous poisoning.

Clinical comment

The treatment and management of salicylate poisoning is well displayed in this patient. The treating team must first consider salicylate poisoning as a diagnosis, and clues to the diagnosis were the mixed acid–base disorder together with impaired renal function and a relatively low blood glucose level. The mildly elevated temperature of 37.4°C and subtle ECG changes are non-specific features, but could retrospectively point towards salicylate poisoning.

Treatment is based around the five well-established principles of toxicological management:

1 Resuscitation: this occurs independently of the cause, and was rapidly instituted in this circumstance.
2 Risk assessment: the clinical effects were striking, in that the patient was unconscious and there was a profound metabolic acidosis. Whatever the toxin, it had exerted a significant effect upon this patient. If an ingested dose can be calculated, toxic effects appear at ingested doses greater than 150 mg/kg of body weight. This can assist clinicians with performing a risk assessment.
3 Prevent absorption: the administration of activated charcoal is recommended for certain toxins if it can be given within 1–2 hours of the ingestion. In the case of salicylate poisoning, it is recommended that charcoal be given up to 8 hours following ingestion, and should be given repeatedly if levels continue to rise.
4 Enhance elimination: salicylic acid has a low pKa of 3.5, and so urinary alkalinisation enhances salicylate excretion from the kidneys. Haemodialysis is effective in removing salicylates from the circulation, but is reserved for severe toxicity (as in this case)

and levels that are rising despite the institution of alkalinisation therapy.

5 Antidote: there is no antidote for salicylates; hence the principle of administering an antidote is not applicable in this case.

There are a number of parameters that suggest that this could be classified as a severe overdose: an altered level of consciousness, significant acid–base disturbance, renal impairment, and a high initial salicylate level.

In anticipation of the need for haemodialysis, a wide-bore multi-lumen vascular catheter is inserted into the right femoral vein. Urinary alkalinisation continues, and the emergency team waits for a bed in the intensive care unit to become available.

Physiology comment

In acetylsalicylic acid poisoning, infusion of sodium bicarbonate is a treatment option that will go some way to buffering the acid addition to the body. Sodium bicarbonate also has the additional effect of increasing the pH of urine, which in turn increases the elimination of salicylate through the urinary system. Most drugs at physiological pH exist partly as undissociated molecules. The extent of dissociation is a function of the ionisation (which is described by the acid dissociation constant, K_a) of the drug and the pH of the fluid in which it is dissolved. Dissociation constants are expressed in the form of their negative logarithm or pK_a. Hence, the stronger an acid the lower its pK_a. As acetylsalicylic acid has an acid dissociation constant of 3.5 at 25°C, it means that it will be only weakly or partially dissociated in the plasma. As the ionisation of a weak acid is increased in an alkaline environment, alkalinisation of the urine will increase the amount of free dissociated acetylsalicylic acid present in the tubular fluid. This traps or retains acetylsalicylic acid in the tubular lumen, as the dissociated acid is less able to pass across the luminal membrane and be reabsorbed back into the peritubular capillaries. In summary, alkalinisation of the urine produces a tubular environment that promotes dissociation of the weak acid, limiting reabsorption, and therefore promotes urinary excretion. Haemodialysis can also be used to enhance the removal of the salicylate from the plasma. Haemodialysis is used in patients with significantly high salicylate blood levels, significant neurotoxicity, renal failure, or pulmonary oedema. Haemodialysis also has the advantage of restoring electrolyte and acid–base abnormalities.

03:27 hours

The patient is transferred to ICU, and haemodialysis commences immediately.

Epilogue

Haemodialysis continued for 24 hours until the salicylate level dropped and the acid–base abnormalities were corrected. The patient was kept sedated until the haemodialysis was completed. The patient woke up and was successfully extubated, and he was then able to tell the ICU staff that he had been feeling depressed and drank a bottle of vodka and ingested the two full boxes of aspirin that were in the bathroom cupboard. The 200 × 300 mg tablets equated to 60 grams of aspirin ingested—a very significant ingestion. The patient recovered fully from this impulsive but potentially fatal event.

Tips

- All patients with reduced levels of consciousness, regardless of the ultimate cause, should be treated the same initially, with clinical staff focusing on keeping them alive through management of their airway, breathing, and circulation.
- The 12-lead ECG is an important prognostic tool in assessing the poisoned patient.
- For expert advice in managing complex poisonings, seek telephone advice from experienced toxicologists at poison information centres.
- The principles of the toxicology risk assessment can be applied in any overdose and can organise the diagnostic and management process logically.

References and further reading

1 Casaletto, J.J. Differential diagnosis of metabolic acidosis. *Emerg Med Clin N Am* 2005; 23: 771–87.
2 Dargan, P.I., Wallace, C.I. & Jones, A.L. An evidence based flowchart to guide the management of acute salicylate (aspirin) overdose. *Emerg Med J* 2002; 19: 206–9.
3 Erickson, T.B., Thompson, T.M. & Lu, J.J. The approach to the patient with an unknown overdose. *Emerg Med Clin N Am* 2007; 25: 249–81.

4   O'Malley, G.F. Emergency department management of the salicylate-poisoned patient. *Emerg Med Clin N Am* May 2007; 25 (2): 333–46.
5   Proudfoot, A.T., Krenzelok, E.P. & Vale, J.A. Position paper on urine alkalinization. *Clinical Toxicology* 2004; 42 (1): 1–26.
6   Merck & Co., Inc. *The Merck Manual Online Library*. Acid–base disorders. <www.merck.com/mmpe/sec12/ch157/ch157b.html> accessed 12 Feb 2009.

Case review

Basic science questions

1   An increased anion gap indicates which of the following?
   A   Excess unmeasured anions in solution
   B   A lactic acidosis
   C   Respiratory compensation
   D   Renal compensation
   E   Metabolic alkalosis

2   The respiratory alkalosis that often develops in cases of salicylate poising is due to which of the following?
   A   Direct stimulation of the respiratory centre
   B   Loss of acid through the kidney
   C   An elevated anion gap
   D   Reduced lung compliance
   E   An increase in TLC

3   Which statement concerning pKa is most correct?
   A   pKa is a measure for comparing the relative strengths of acids
   B   pKa of an acid is a measure of the free hydrogen ion concentration
   C   pKa decreases with temperature
   D   pKa is increased during diabetic ketoacidosis
   E   pKa of plasma is elevated during respiratory distress

Clinical questions

1   Match the following clinical condition with the corresponding acid–base disorder.
   A   A 57-year-old male presents with severe central crushing chest pain, profuse sweating, and a blood pressure of 80/50.
   B   A 68-year-old female with emphysema presents acutely breathless and with a reduced level of consciousness.
   C   A 32-year-old female on diuretics presents with two episodes of syncope.
   D   A 23-year-old male presents with cyanosis and has consolidation in the lower lobe of his left lung.

E A 78-year-old male with renal failure presents with sepsis from his peritoneal dialysis catheter.
  (i) Acute on chronic metabolic acidosis
  (ii) Metabolic alkalosis
  (iii) Acute on chronic respiratory acidosis
  (iv) Acute metabolic acidosis
  (v) Acute respiratory alkalosis

2 Which of the following conditions is least likely to produce a metabolic acidosis?
  A Multiple major trauma with hypovolaemic shock
  B Ingestion of formaldehyde
  C Tension pneumothorax
  D Severe acute exacerbation of asthma
  E Acute renal failure

3 Which of the following treatments is not recommended for salicylate poisoning?
  A Activated charcoal
  B Forced saline diuresis
  C Potassium replacement
  D Administration of sodium bicarbonate
  E Prostaglandin administration

Appendix
Map of cases and topics

Case	Biomedical topic	Case summary	Pathology and physiology	Investigations	Clinical issues	Acid–base balance
1	Diuretic use	Teenaged female using diuretics to maintain weight has dizzy spells	Control of blood pressure and postural hypotension The body fluid compartments Dehydration and hypovolaemia Homeostasis Hydration state and reviewing electrolyte values Thiazide diuretics	U&E FBC ECG	Syncope	
2	Hypernatraemia 1	Elderly lady with heat-related illness and fall	Assessing renal function Hypernatraemia Regulation of Na balance	U&E CK	Syncope Heat stroke Rhabdomyolysis Fractured neck of femur	Metabolic acidosis Renal and respiratory compensation
3	Hypernatraemia 2	Small bowel obstruction	Electrolyte and fluid alterations brought about by vomiting	U&E X-rays	Dehydration Bowel obstruction	

Case	Biomedical topic	Case summary	Pathology and physiology	Investigations	Clinical issues	Acid–base balance
4	Hyponatraemia	Vomiting young child ultimately diagnosed a UTI	Vomiting reflex Paradoxical aciduria	U&E Urine microbiology	Assessment and management of the unwell febrile child Urinary tract infection	Metabolic alkalosis with a co-existing volume depletion
5	Isotonic volume loss	Ruptured AAA with hypovolaemic shock	Cardiovascular responses to hypovolaemic shock Fluid shifts Colloid versus crystalloid therapy Acute renal success and failure	U&E FBC COAGS ABG Anion gap	Resuscitation of shock Ruptured AAA	Lactic acidosis
6	DKA and hypovolaemia	Viral illness in IDDM acute presentation	DKA Volume and potassium balance	ABG U&E Glucose FBC	Acutely unwell diabetic with ketoacidosis Potassium management	Metabolic acidosis

Case	Biomedical topic	Case summary	Pathology and physiology	Investigations	Clinical issues	Acid–base balance
7	Hypokalaemia	Elderly male with CHF on frusemide and oral potassium	Pulmonary oedema Congestive cardiac failure β-type natriuretic factor Potassium balance and hypokalaemia	U&E BNP Troponin	Exacerbation and precipitants of congestive cardiac failure	
8	Elevated anion gap, hypocalcaemia	Pancreatitis	Pancreatitis Introduce the ideas of anion gap and base deficit Hypocalcaemia.	Lipase FBC U&E Ca ABG Anion gap	Undifferentiated abdominal pain Appropriate use of investigations	Metabolic acidosis
9	Respiratory acidosis	Asthma attack during excessive smoke in atmosphere	Asthma Respiratory acidosis and compensation	ABG	Management of acute dyspnoea Classification of asthma Airway management	Respiratory acidosis

Case	Biomedical topic	Case summary	Pathology and physiology	Investigations	Clinical issues	Acid–base balance
10	Salicylate overdose	Toxicology	Mixed disorders Respiratory alkalosis and metabolic acidosis Acidosis and potassium balance Anion gap	ABG U&E Serum salicylate level	Toxicology Management of reduced level of consciousness	Mixed acid–base disorder

Answers

Case 1 review

Level 1: Basic science questions

1 A
2 C
3 E

Level 2: Clinical questions

1 **A** (iv)
  B (iii)
  C (v)
  D (i)
  E (ii)
2 C There appear to be no concerning features; so this patient could be discharged with advice to maintain an appropriate fluid intake. The other options could all potentially have serious underlying conditions: A—possible underlying cardiac ischaemia, B—ectopic pregnancy, D—intracerebral event (or migraine), and E—possible pulmonary embolism.
3 B Normal saline is a crystalloid, is cost-effective, and is entirely appropriate for rehydration.

Case 2 review

Level 1: Basic science questions

1 A
2 C
3 D

Level 2: Clinical questions

1 **A** (i)
  B (iv)
  C (ii)
  D (iii) Refer to the dehydration table in Case 1 on page 7.
2 A 0.9% saline is the most physiological of all these fluids, and hence distributes to the interstitial and intracellular spaces.
3 B heat exhaustion

Case 3 review

Level 1: Basic science questions

1 A
2 E
3 C

Level 2: Clinical questions

1 **A** (ii)
  B (v)
  C (iv) (CT renal colic protocol in particular)
  D (i)
  E (iii)
2 D Metoclopramide, as this agent has an anti-emetic effect by having prokinetic effect upon gut smooth muscle. In the event of a distal obstruction, this would be obviously counterproductive and could make the proximal bowel dilatation worse.
3 A, D dry: these are features of hypoperfusion and dehydration.
  B, C wet: these are features of pulmonary and interstitial oedema, serious but common consequences of fluid overload.

Case 4 review

Level 1: Basic science questions

1 A
2 C
3 E

Level 2: Clinical questions

1   **A** (iv)
    B (ii)
    C (i)
    D (iii)
2   B   5% dextrose. This is a hypotonic fluid once the dextrose is metabolised, leaving just free water being infused, and its use can lead to dangerous hyponatraemia. This is a risk with any intravenous fluid; so electrolytes must be closely monitored and infusion amounts regularly reviewed and adjusted.
3   **A** (iii)
    B (ii)
    C (i)
    D (iv)

Case 5 review

Level 1: Basic science questions

1   B
2   A
3   C

Level 2: Clinical questions

1   D   Aortic aneurysms are rare to those under the age of 50.
2   **A** (iv) This is unsurvivable.
    B (i)
    C (ii) This patient has the best chance of surviving an operation and the post-operative period. Fluids should not be given at this stage because vital organs are being perfused—the patient needs a rapid transit to theatre.
    D (iii) Resuscitation should commence, and if there is a response the patient may have a chance of survival, but mortality is high. If there is no response to resuscitation then palliation may be the best option.

Case 6 review

Level 1: Basic science questions

1 D
2 C
3 A

Level 2: Clinical questions

1 **A** (i)
  B (iii) This has an element of acute-on-chronic acidosis, as evidenced by an elevated bicarbonate in compensation. The patient probably has an exacerbation of chronic obstructive pulmonary disease (COPD).
  C (iv)
  D (ii)
2 C With a metabolic acidosis, hyperventilation would be expected by producing a low pCO_2 to compensate. However, in severe cases where the patient is obtunded, this may not be possible.
3 D In a dehydrated patient with significant electrolyte and acid–base abnormalities there is no clinical indication or evidence for using such a fluid. All other fluids listed may have a role at different stages of the resuscitation.

Case 7 review

Level 1: Basic science questions

1 A
2 D
3 B

Level 2: Clincial questions

1 C Verapamil. Calcium channel blockers are negative inotropes and can exacerbate heart failure. Interestingly, β-blockers (which include carvedilol) were long thought to be contra-indicated for similar reasons, but studies have shown that they in fact improve survival.
2 E Each of these conditions can exacerbate heart failure.
3 B Frusemide. It does have a role in managing heart failure, but plays little role in the management of acute pulmonary oedema.

Case 8 review

Level 1: Basic science questions

1 E
2 D
3 E

Level 2: Clinical questions

1 **A** (v)
   B (ii)
   C (i)
   D (iii)
   E (iv) Note that conditions (i) to (iv) are surgical emergencies and require urgent referral. Cholangitis and gallstone pancreatitis require urgent ERCP (endoscopic retrograde cholangiopancreatography) by an experienced gastroenterologist.
2 D All of the others are recognised causes. Note that in approximately 20% of cases no cause can be identified ('idiopathic').
3 D Diarrhoea. This leads to a loss of bicarbonate from the gut (as well as other metabolites in differing proportions). Causes of a normal anion gap acidosis can be remembered by the mnemonic HARDUP: Hyperalimentation, Acetazolamide, Renal tubular acidosis and renal insufficiency, Diarrhoea and diuretics, Ureteroenterostomy, and Pancreatic fistula.

Case 9 review

Level 1: Basic science questions

1 D
2 A
3 E

Level 2: Clinical questions

1 **A** (i)
   B (iv)
   C (iii)
   D (ii)

2 C Leukotriene receptor antagonists have no role in the management of acute asthma. Non-invasive ventilation may have a role but its use must be constantly assessed for efficacy.

Case 10 review

Level 1: Basic science questions

1 A
2 A
3 A

Level 2: Clinical questions

1 **A** (iv)
 B (iii)
 C (ii)
 D (v)
 E (i)
2 D Severe asthma tends to produce an acute respiratory acidosis rather than a metabolic acidosis (but, as was seen in Case 9, it can co-exist).
3 B Diuresis was once recommended therapy but has since been found to be potentially dangerous and not to improve outcomes.

Index